The Cortisol Reset Plan

The Cortisol Reset Plan

THE **COMPLETE GUIDE** TO BALANCING YOUR HORMONES, REVERSING WEIGHT GAIN, AND RESTORING NERVOUS SYSTEM HEALTH

MARINA WRIGHT, FDNP

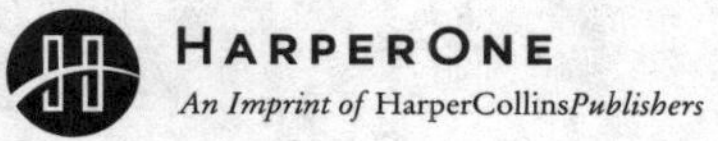
HARPERONE
An Imprint of HarperCollins*Publishers*

This book contains advice and information relating to health care. It should be used to supplement rather than replace the advice of your doctor or another trained health professional. If you know or suspect you have a health problem, it is recommended that you seek your physician's advice before embarking on any medical program or treatment. All efforts have been made to assure the accuracy of the information contained in this book as of the date of publication. This publisher and the author disclaim liability for any medical outcomes that may occur as a result of applying the methods suggested in this book.

The material on linked sites referenced in this book is the author's own. HarperCollins disclaims all liability that may result from the use of the material contained at those sites. All such material is supplemental and not part of the book. The author reserves the right to close the website in her sole discretion at any time.

 For information, address HarperCollins Publishers, 195 Broadway, New York, NY 10007. In Europe, HarperCollins Publishers, Macken House, 39/40 Mayor Street Upper, Dublin 1, D01 C9W8, Ireland.

HarperCollins books may be purchased for educational, business, or sales promotional use. For information, please email the Special Markets Department at SPsales@harpercollins.com.

harpercollins.com

ORIGINALLY PUBLISHED IN THE UNITED KINGDOM IN 2025 BY VERMILLION.

FIRST US EDITION

Designed by Leah Carlson-Stanisic and Yvonne Chan

Library of Congress Cataloging-in-Publication Data has been applied for.

ISBN 978-0-06-343627-5

25 26 27 28 29 LBC 5 4 3 2 1

To my mother—brave, kind, and forever in my heart.

Contents

Introduction

I am not afraid of storms, for I am learning how to sail my ship.

—LOUISA MAY ALCOTT

If the title of this book has piqued your interest, you're likely on a personal journey toward what I call a state of *optimal health*: a strong body and a calm mind. A body that feels good to live in: pain-free, moving with ease, at a healthy weight, and energized to allow you to enjoy an active life. And a mind that's resilient and at peace, free from the weight of chronic anxiety, overthinking, or emotional pain, and that allows you to face every day with confidence and a sense of control.

I know this might sound too good to be true, but deep down, I think you already sense that this state is not only possible, it's your birthright! You sense this because within you lies an innate wisdom, and a natural ability to heal and thrive. Yet, like so many of us on this journey, you probably feel overwhelmed, disheartened, and unsure how to access your inner potential.

Despite all your efforts, your symptoms persist: anxiety, chronic fatigue, chronic pain, hormonal imbalances, autoimmune issues, weight gain, brain fog, digestive problems such as irritable bowel syndrome (IBS), or just a sense that something is still "off."

You've likely tried almost "everything" by now, from conventional methods like doctor visits, talk therapy, medications, diets, and the general advice to "just eat better and exercise more," to more "alternative" approaches such as naturopathy, herbs and supplements, detox programs, acupuncture, and more. While these may have provided some temporary relief, I expect they haven't delivered the *lasting* healing or that optimal state of health and well-being you long for.

I know exactly how you feel because I've been in your shoes. I've experienced the physical and emotional pain that can leave you desperate for relief.

My Story

When I was in my mid-twenties, after completing my law degree in Spain, I moved to London to take on an exciting corporate job. I met my partner, whom I later married, built a great group of friends, and spent weekends exploring the city, immersing myself in new places and experiences. From the outside, I probably projected an image of success, health, calm, and happiness. However, beneath the surface, I was far from healthy or happy.

During my work breaks, I often found myself in tears in the office bathroom because of the overwhelming pressure of my job. I struggled with a complicated relationship with food and exercise, fighting hard to maintain a body shape that I believed would make me liked and accepted. Emotionally, I was still suffering from the loss of my mother to a long and traumatic battle with cancer, a battle that started when I was just a kid. Mentally, I was always worrying about the future, ruminating about the past, and pushing myself to do more because, surely, I thought, I wasn't trying hard enough to be better. Deep inside, I thought I was broken.

My high-functioning anxiety gradually worsened over time, leaving me less able to cope and leading to panic attacks in completely normal and safe situations, like on the London Underground, in the middle of a work meeting, or even when trying to fall asleep at night. If you have had panic attacks, you know how scary and debilitating they can be, and how they just make your life smaller and smaller as you try to avoid anything that might trigger them.

You can see how far my mind was from calm! My body, on the other hand, had always been very strong and healthy . . . up until my move to London.

My physical health began to deteriorate and I didn't understand why. It started with skin rashes and acne, but then it got progressively worse with more and more symptoms: constant bloating, digestive issues, fatigue, and irregular menstrual cycles, eventually leading to my periods disappearing for months at a time. Multiple doctor visits led to multiple drug prescriptions: antibiotics for my skin and gut issues, selective serotonin reuptake inhibitors (SSRIs) to manage anxiety, and birth control to regulate my cycles. My symptoms did improve, but they never fully resolved.

A couple of years later, when my husband and I decided to try for a baby, I faced a long struggle with infertility, which eventually led us to pursue fertility treatments. I was very lucky to be able to conceive and deliver a beautiful baby boy. However, without warning, I plunged into the depths of postpartum depression just days after my son's birth.

My anxiety came back with a vengeance as I struggled with the overwhelming responsibility of caring for a newborn. At the time, we had recently relocated to New York, and my husband, who had a demanding job that required long working hours and frequent travel, often had to leave me alone in our tiny apartment during one of the hottest summers the city had seen in years.

Day after day, I found myself isolated in that apartment, the air-conditioning my only relief from the outdoor heat. I felt alone and unsupported, but even worse, I felt guilty and completely inadequate. I was 100 percent convinced that there was something very wrong with me and I didn't deserve to be happy. Looking back, I realize this was my rock bottom.

Desperate for help, I reached out to my obstetrician, but he failed to return my call. Instead, he left a prescription for Xanax (an anxiety-reducing medication) at reception for me to pick up and told me to take it whenever I felt too overwhelmed. When I returned for my 6-week checkup, he did all the necessary physical exams, but he never asked about my state of mind, my anxiety, or my mental health.

Despite all these challenges, I consider myself lucky because hitting rock bottom proved to be the catalyst for real transformation. I wish I could tell you that I had an epiphany or went through a dark night of the soul that "enlightened" me and changed everything overnight, but the reality is that it took much longer than that.

The first few months after my son was born were focused on taking care of my body and incorporating a few *simple* habits that I could easily follow while looking after him. These habits gave me a sense of control over my life and, little by little, I started to feel better—physically, mentally, and emotionally—each day.

It was the following months and years that brought real transformation, though. I left the corporate world to immerse myself in studying the mind-body connection and explore fields like nutrition, psychology, biology, neuroscience, and the intricate workings of the nervous system. Understanding how the nervous system influences the stress response and overall health became key to my healing, helping me connect the dots between mental and physical well-being. I gradually adopted a new approach to both diet and lifestyle that provided results that had seemed unattainable at the beginning of my healing journey.

My menstrual cycles became regular, my persistent gut issues slowly resolved, my skin cleared up, I could fall asleep easily and stay asleep all night, and my panic attacks became less and less frequent until they eventually disappeared. I stopped obsessing about food and exercise because I was eating a nourishing diet that left me satisfied and helped me to achieve my optimal weight without really trying. I conceived my second son and, this time, I fully embraced the first few months without the weight of postpartum depression. I felt a sense of calm and confidence as a mother that I hadn't known before.

Establishing my own practice and later developing online programs allowed me to help others struggling with similar symptoms. Through years of clinical practice and personal experience, I refined a progressive, step-by-step method that serves as the foundation for the book you now hold in your hands.

My story and challenges taught me a few crucial lessons that I hope will help you in your own path toward rebuilding your health and vitality:

- **You are not broken:** Your body wants to heal and has a natural ability to do so once you harness the powerful mind-body connection.
- **You are in the driver's seat of your health journey:** No one else is responsible for your well-being but you. While this may seem daunting, it's also very liberating and empowering because YOU are the one who has the power to change. This doesn't mean you have to do it alone; your health providers, your family, and your friends are all there to guide and support you. But, ultimately, only you have the power to take charge of your healing.
- **Small habits have big impact:** Small habits might seem insignificant at first, but when practiced consistently over the long term, they can create powerful changes.

About This Book

The Cortisol Reset Plan is your road map to unlocking the mind-body connection for lasting health, and to being able to meet your days with the energy you deserve to have! Packed with practical tools, it will guide you to reconnect with your body, rewire your brain, and build the resilience you need to thrive.

This book is for you if you:

- struggle with persistent or recurrent symptoms such as constant fatigue, poor sleep, weight gain, brain fog, premenstrual syndrome (PMS), hormonal imbalances, chronic pain, autoimmune issues, or digestive issues like IBS;
- experience mood swings, anxiety or depression, or just don't feel like yourself;
- have tried addressing your symptoms but haven't found lasting relief;
- suspect that stress may be at the root of your health challenges;
- want a step-by-step guide with simple, actionable tools to help you not only heal but also achieve optimal health, a strong body, and a calm mind.

The book is divided into three parts.

Part I: The Mind-Body Connection explores the whys and hows. It leans more scientific, but I've made sure to present it in a way that's accessible and easy to follow. Understanding what is happening and why your body and mind are doing what they are doing will allow you to have a lot more compassion toward yourself, and your newfound knowledge will make applying the five steps of the Cortisol Reset Plan much more effective.

You'll also find two questionnaires in this section, designed to help you assess where you are right now and give you a baseline for tracking your progress throughout the plan.

Part I will help you connect the dots, and I promise you'll have plenty of "aha" moments!

Part II: The Cortisol Reset Plan introduces a five-step framework to build stress resilience, reverse your symptoms, and achieve a state of optimal health: that strong body and calm mind we've been talking about. The five steps are:

1. Eat a Nutrient-Dense Diet
2. Balance Your Blood Sugar
3. Regulate Your Circadian Rhythm
4. Exercise for Mind and Body Health
5. Build Psychological Resilience and Well-Being

The ultimate goal of these steps is to expand your "stress bucket" capacity—your ability to tolerate and recover from stress. We'll achieve this by:

- Reducing *physical* stressors that often go unnoticed but overwhelm your system, such as blood sugar imbalances or chronic inflammation.
- Reducing "faulty" *perceived* stressors by improving how your brain interprets signals from the environment and from what is going on inside your body.
- Improving the mind-body connection through the nervous system using somatic (body-based) practices (like body awareness, mindful movement, and breathwork) to help regulate emotional and physical responses.
- Rewiring your brain's responses, creating more adaptive reactions to stress.
- Building your metabolic reserves and energy, which enhances your body's ability to cope with stressors and improves resilience over time.

Part III: The Cortisol Reset Recipes will provide you with a variety of meal ideas for breakfast, lunch, snacks, and dinner, as well as some gut-healing recipes, all designed to help you easily put into practice everything you will learn in Steps One (Eat a Nutrient-Dense Diet) and Two (Balance Your Blood Sugar). I've created these recipes by applying the guidelines from both steps, transforming them into simple, easy-to-make meals.

At the back of the book are some appendices, which offer additional resources to support your healing journey, including at-home testing options, simple ways to reduce your exposure to toxins, as well as information on adaptogens and other nutritional compounds that can enhance your resilience to stress.

While grounded in scientific research, this book is definitely not an academic paper. Instead, it's designed to be an accessible read that offers practical tips you can start implementing straight away. My general recommendation is for you to read through Part I so you understand the mind-body connection, then focus on each step in Part II for *1 or 2 weeks* before moving on to the next. However, you might find that the habits in some steps are easier to implement than others or that you're already familiar with some of the practices and habits of a particular step, allowing you to move through that step more quickly. On the other hand, you might need extra time in a particular step or life can get busy, slowing your pace, and that is absolutely fine, too. Feel free to adapt the timeline to suit you and your learning style. This is your own healing journey.

Gradually integrating the habits from each step, and practicing them consistently, will yield more long-term benefits than overwhelming yourself with too many changes at once.

To help you track your progress, at the end of each step, I've included a checklist with the most important habits to integrate. Once these habits feel natural and almost automatic to you, you can confidently move on to the next step.

I also recommend redoing the questionnaires from Part I at the end of each step. It's a helpful way to reflect on your progress and notice any changes in how you're feeling—physically, mentally, and emotionally.

My hope is that this book becomes your go-to guide, a resource you can revisit time and time again for support on your personal journey to lasting health and well-being.

Let's begin!

Part I

The Mind-Body Connection

Understanding the Nervous System

We suffer more often in imagination than in reality.
—SENECA

First, thank you for turning to this first chapter. I know it's tempting to skip straight to the plan in Part II, but as I mentioned in the Introduction, learning about the mind-body connection will make integrating the five steps much more effective. After all, long-term healing begins with understanding your nervous system because it connects your mind (your thoughts, emotions, and cognition) with your body (which includes things like hormone regulation, digestion, immune response, heart rate, metabolism, breathing, muscle movement, and more). Through this connection, the nervous system plays a key role in shaping both your mental and physical health. It's the cornerstone of the mind-body connection.

To understand your nervous system, you need to think about what its main motivation is for doing what it does, and that is to keep you *safe*.

How the Nervous System Works

Your nervous system is made up of both the central nervous system (the brain and spinal cord) and the peripheral nervous system (the network of nerves outside the brain and spinal cord). You can think of it as your body's *surveillance system,* constantly sending, receiving, and interpreting information to answer the question *Is this safe?*

The central nervous system is the processing and command center, while the peripheral nervous system connects the central nervous system to the rest of your body, relaying messages in both directions.

The peripheral nervous system is divided into two main divisions based on the direction information flows:

1. Sensory (Afferent) Division

   This division carries information from your body to your brain—helping your brain understand what's happening both outside and inside you. It gathers information through:

   - Exteroception, using your five senses—sight, hearing, taste, smell, and touch—to detect the external world.
   - Interoception, which monitors signals from inside your body, such as hunger, thirst, body temperature, pain, inflammation, blood sugar levels, or the need to use the bathroom.

› Proprioception and vestibular input, which together provide information about your body's position, movement, and balance, helping your brain know where you are in space and how you're moving.

2. Motor (Efferent) Division

   This division carries commands from your brain to your body, telling your muscles, organs, and glands what to do. It has two main branches:

   › Somatic Motor System: Controls *voluntary* movements, like picking something up, walking, or smiling.

   › Autonomic Nervous System (ANS): Controls *involuntary* functions you don't consciously think about, such as your heart beating, digestion, breathing, and blood pressure. The ANS itself splits into two parts:

     – Sympathetic Nervous System: Activates "fight or flight," which is a key part of the body's overall stress response, preparing you to react quickly to perceived threats.

     – Parasympathetic Nervous System: Promotes "rest and digest" functions, helping the body relax and recover after stress.

So, your brain receives sensory information from both outside and inside your body. If it interprets any of that information as a threat, it activates the motor divisions to respond. Some responses are voluntary—like moving away from danger—but many are involuntary and are automatically controlled by the ANS, such as *the stress response* (which we will discuss shortly).

The responses are the outputs, which are the changes that help the body adapt to the perceived threat, ultimately aiming to keep you safe.

Inputs (environment and internal signals) → brain interpretation of the signals → outputs (responses to allow adaptation)

It sounds like the nervous system should be your best ally and, in many ways, it truly is. After all, its primary goal is to keep you alive! However, it can sometimes become a liability when it becomes overactive or hypervigilant, or when the messages sent to the brain get fuzzy or are misinterpreted—leading it to see threats everywhere and triggering the stress response again and again. This dysregulation is taxing on both the mind and body, leading to allostatic load, which is "the wear and tear on the body" that accumulates when exposed to repeated or chronic stress, and a concept called *allostatic load*, which we will discuss in detail shortly.[1]

So, why does the nervous system become dysregulated? Our nervous system is fundamentally the same now as it was in our ancestors, hundreds of thousands of years ago. However, the number and type of threats we face today are different from those our ancestors encountered. Back then, our bodies were designed to respond to *occasional* dangers, like predators or environmental hazards. But today, we're bombarded *hourly* with an overwhelming amount of modern stressors, such as work pressure, mortgages, traffic, information overload (overwhelming news, angry people on social media), environmental toxins, ultra-processed foods, lack of sleep, and more. The nervous system was built for a different world, one that no longer exists for most modern humans, and it struggles to distinguish these modern stressors from true *life-or-death threats.*

> **Your nervous system was wired for a different world, one without the constant hustle of modern stressors.**

WHAT ARE STRESSORS?

When you think of stress, you probably think about the usual culprits such as work pressures, losing a loved one, relationship challenges, or financial struggles. But stress is a much broader concept than that, and much of it is "hidden"; it's below your conscious awareness.

To give you a few examples: Stress can be present in the sleep-deprived new parent, the office worker facing an important deadline, the couple about to get married, the health-conscious person doing cold plunges, the person eating an ultra-processed food diet, the person on a very restrictive diet, the student preparing for exams, the teenager going on their first date, the marathon runner, the commuter navigating daily traffic, or the person dealing with an infection.

Stress shows up in multiple ways and it's an intrinsic part of the human experience. It's not something that we can avoid and, in fact, certain stressors are beneficial because they help us grow, adapt, build resilience, and even boost health (think exercise, cold exposure, fasting, or mentally challenging activities like learning new skills, for example). However, it is also true that certain stressors create physiological, behavioral, emotional, and cognitive changes that can lead to physical and mental health issues.

We can label a stressor as "good" or "toxic" depending on how much control we have over it and the resources (energy) and capacity (resilience) we have in place for coping with it.[2] You are going to see the words "energy" and "resilience" a lot in this book because they both hold the key to your healing.

While people face different events or stressors, they respond with the same set of physiological changes—this is called the "stress response," and we will discuss what it entails in detail shortly. From the perspective of the stressor, it doesn't even matter whether the event is "good" (marriage, date, promotion) or "toxic" (illness, argument, deadline). However, the degree of threat will determine the magnitude of the response.

Stress isn't exclusive to humans either. It's a universal experience shared by animals and plants alike. After all, the demands of survival affect all living beings. For example, an animal may experience stress when facing a predator, and a plant can face stress due to factors like extreme weather conditions or nutrient deficiencies. What sets humans apart from animals and plants, though, is our unique ability to *perceive* and anticipate stressors that may not even exist in reality but are imagined, residing "in our heads." This subjective nature of stress adds a layer of complexity to the human experience.

Sound familiar? Think about when you ask your partner or kids to call when they reach their destination, but hours pass without a word. As time goes on, your brain starts anticipating, ruminating, and preparing itself for the worst-case scenario. Your brain does that because it hates uncertainty, but by doing so, it's unnecessarily preparing your body to face a threat that exists only in your imagination. Later, when your loved one finally calls, you learn that their phone ran out of battery, and you feel relieved and also a bit silly for worrying unnecessarily. The narrative you created was imagined and yet your body reacted as if it were 100 percent real. The human mind is arguably the most potent trigger of unnecessary stress responses.

We'll look at stressors in more detail in the next chapter, but these can be broadly categorized into two groups:

1. **Perceived (psychological) stressors:** These can be real, but as we've seen, they can also be imagined—and each person perceives them differently depending on their past experiences, genetic makeup, and current levels of stress. They are psychological and emotional, and arguably the most damaging for our long-term health. Examples include relationship problems, financial strain, work pressures, unresolved childhood trauma, and job insecurity. Sociopolitical stressors, such as discrimination or inequality, play a significant role as well.
2. **Physical stressors:** These are an actual threat to our survival; they are not "imagined." Examples include lack of sleep, chronic inflammation, nutrient deficiencies, physical injuries, prolonged exposure to environmental toxins, chronic illness, ongoing physical overwork, blood sugar imbalances, and more.

The way each of us reacts to stimuli is influenced by our genes, past experiences, childhood trauma, and our current physical and mental health.

Once your brain *identifies* a threat (real or imagined), it triggers the stress response to adapt, cope, or face the threat.

The Stress Response

To thrive, humans, and all living things, must maintain a *stable internal environment* in which the cells of the body live and survive.[3] This means keeping things like temperature, pH, oxygen, carbon dioxide, glucose, and hormone levels within a tight range. This stable environment is known as *homeostasis*, a state that is constantly challenged by internal and external threats or stressors.

When this balance is threatened, the body activates a set of adaptive responses to *restore* homeostasis. These are allostatic responses, and I will discuss allostasis in more detail shortly. For now, let's focus on a key allostatic response—the stress response.

The stress response involves the ANS and the hypothalamic-pituitary-adrenal (HPA) axis (the system that connects the brain and adrenal glands to release the "stress hormone" cortisol).

As we mentioned earlier, the ANS has two branches: the sympathetic nervous system (SNS), which activates the "fight-or-flight" response, and the parasympathetic nervous system (PNS), which helps the body "rest and digest" once the threat has passed.

Let's walk through a scenario that shows the stress response in action. Imagine you're hiking through the woods, when, suddenly, you spot a bear. In a split second, upon perceiving a threat of a predator, the first phase of the stress response (also called the short-term stress response) kicks in with the release of epinephrine (known more commonly as adrenaline) and norepinephine (noradrenaline). These are hormone-neurotransmitters that flood your brain and peripheral tissues, triggering the fight-or-flight response and preparing you for *immediate* action. Your heart rate, blood pressure, and breathing increase to deliver more oxygen to your muscles and brain to help you run or think of a way to escape from the bear. Additionally, glucose is released into the bloodstream to provide *energy*.

If the threat is not resolved and the stressor persists, the second phase of the stress response activates the HPA axis, which ramps up within minutes to sustain the body's alert state after the immediate fight-or-flight response. This is called the long-term stress response, and it involves the release of cortisol, which helps your body *prolong* the stress response. Cortisol has many overlapping effects with adrenaline and noradrenaline, especially having the same goal to increase energy by mobilizing glucose, fats, and amino acids, but the difference is that cortisol effects last a lot longer (adrenaline might last for just seconds, but cortisol lasts for minutes or even hours).

Throughout all of this, you would be noticing several things happening in your body. You might feel that your heart is racing and your breathing is fast and shallow. Your muscles might feel tense and your hands clammy. Your stomach might feel queasy and your mouth dry.

Now notice how all those sensations are familiar to you—even though you've probably never been chased by a bear! That's because the stress response is a generic reaction to any threat identified by your brain, whether it's encountering a wild animal, your toddler having a meltdown in the supermarket, or preparing for a public speech.

Once the bear leaves or you get to safety, your PNS takes over, calming things down and slowly bringing your body back to its normal state. Your heart rate slows, your blood pressure drops, and your body returns to a more balanced state, hence why it is also known as "rest and digest."

While the stress response is critical for adapting to internal and external challenges, the body's ability to *recover* and return to homeostasis after the threat has passed is just as important. Without recovery, recurrent or chronic activation of the stress response can change it from being adaptive to maladaptive, resulting in negative health consequences over time. (We'll dive into these negative effects in just a moment.)

This is the paradox of the stress response: The response itself might become more damaging than the stressors it is trying to protect you from.

Remember: The effectiveness of the stress response isn't just about how well the body adapts to challenges, but how quickly it can reset and restore balance. Balancing these two processes is essential for long-term resilience and health.

ALLOSTATIC LOAD

To understand how long-term exposure to stress can lead to negative effects on our physical and mental health, we are going to use the allostatic load model introduced by Bruce McEwen and Elliot Stellar in the early 1990s.[4]

Allostasis refers to the body's ability to adjust and change its systems to operate above or below the normal homeostatic range to adapt to stressors. For instance, remember how, as part of the stress response, cortisol temporarily rises above normal levels to help the body cope with a stressor.

In the short term, allostasis is adaptive. However, when threats are too frequent or when the stress response remains turned on when it's no longer needed, the key players involved in allostasis, such as cortisol, adrenaline, noradrenaline, metabolic hormones, and cytokines (proteins that help control the immune system), can produce a wear and tear on the body that has been termed "allostatic load."[5]

Allostatic load refers to the *cumulative* burden that chronic and acute stress places on the body and has been linked to negative physical and psychological health problems. Exactly how stress can lead to poor health outcomes is not fully understood, but it is thought to be a combination of the long-term effects of the overuse of those key players we just mentioned that are involved in allostasis, the "energetic cost" of maintaining the stress response as chronically activated, and changes in brain plasticity.[6] Let's talk a little bit more about the energetic cost of stress.

Your body doesn't have unlimited resources—it has a *limited* energy reserve, like a "budget" that must be allocated to meet various demands. When we deplete this reserve by overspending on allostatic processes, the body has to redirect energy from somewhere else. The progression from allostasis to allostatic load happens when the body spends so much energy managing stress that it doesn't have enough left for other important functions like growth, maintenance, and repair, which are necessary for long-term health and longevity.[7] It makes sense that the body would put on hold things like immune surveillance, digestion, wound healing, waste removal, reproduction, or DNA repair to be able to redirect energy resources for immediate survival needs. However, over the long term, the limitation of energy and resources for growth, maintenance, and repair processes accelerates the gradual breakdown and damage of cells, tissues, and organs in the body, culminating in the onset and progression of disease.

To use the analogy of a bank, it's like repeatedly taking out loans and constantly wasting money (energy/resources) for short-term survival, rather than investing in the long-term health and wellness fund.

> **Remember:** Allostatic load happens when the demands of everyday stressors (emotional and physical) outweigh a person's ability to cope, which shifts allostasis from adaptive to maladaptive. This is due to both the effects of the overuse of allostatic players (like cortisol) and the reallocation of resources from long-term health functions to short-term survival.

Research has shown a clear connection between allostatic load and negative health outcomes. Findings from a systematic review of 267 studies indicated that allostatic load is associated with poorer health outcomes and is linked to:

- hypertension
- cardiovascular disease
- diabetes
- chronic fatigue syndrome (CFS)
- fibromyalgia

- chronic migraines
- reproductive health issues
- periodontal disease
- cancer
- worsening of physical health markers, including higher inflammation, increased body mass index (BMI), poor cholesterol levels, lower bone mineral density, and nutrient deficiencies
- neurological problems, including worsened cognitive function
- mental health conditions, including depression, anxiety, post-traumatic stress disorder (PTSD), and psychotic disorders[8]

The review also mentions that high allostatic load levels are associated with health-damaging lifestyle habits such as poor sleep, lack of exercise, unhealthy diets, alcohol use and dependence, and smoking. These place additional strain on the body, increasing allostatic load. Stress has also been strongly linked to gut problems, such as IBS, inflammatory bowel disease (IBD), and gastroesophageal reflux disease (GERD).[9]

Homeostasis (normal) → Allostasis (adaptation to stressors) → Allostatic Load (failed adaptation to stressors) → Allostatic Overload (adverse health outcomes)

You're probably starting to see why addressing your symptoms in isolation, whether it's fatigue, weight gain, anxiety, sleep issues, autoimmune conditions, digestive problems, or hormonal imbalances, can be short-sighted. These are simply outputs or manifestations of a larger issue that has been building up for years.

True healing begins at the root, by addressing the mind-body connection to build *resilience*, which is your ability to cope with everyday stressors, both emotional and physical, which is exactly what the five steps of the Cortisol Reset Plan are going to help you achieve. This will help you shift from allostatic load toward adaptive allostasis and homeostasis and eliminate chronic stress symptoms, regardless of how they manifest, while decreasing your risk of diseases and premature ageing by directing energy toward growth, repair, and maintenance.

Let's now dive into one of the key players involved in allostasis, the hormone cortisol—the reason you're reading this book! Here we'll learn what it is, what it does and how it plays a dual role in protecting and potentially harming the body.

THE ROLE OF CORTISOL

Cortisol is a glucocorticoid hormone produced by the adrenal glands. We saw earlier that cortisol, along with adrenaline and noradrenaline, ensure the body has the resources it needs to handle a threat or stressor effectively. They do that mainly by increasing energy supply (increasing glucose and fatty acids in the bloodstream) and regulating immune cells and cytokine production. However, cortisol has many functions other than the stress response: It regulates blood pressure, electrolyte balance (minerals like sodium and potassium that support fluid levels, nerve signaling, and muscle function), your metabolism, your immune system, and much more. So, even though it gets a bad rap, we need cortisol, but in just the right amount.

Something that is helpful to understand about cortisol is that the body produces this hormone in two key ways: following a daily pattern and on an ad hoc basis in response to stress. Regarding the daily pattern, in a healthy person, cortisol levels peak when they wake up and then decline steadily throughout the day, with lowest levels at night.

- **Morning:** Cortisol levels usually begin to rise during the early morning hours and peak shortly after you wake up, typically between 6 and 9 a.m. This peak is called the "cortisol awakening response," or CAR, and helps provide the energy needed to start the day.
- **Daytime:** Throughout the day, cortisol levels gradually decrease, although ad hoc extra release of cortisol might be needed (in response to stress) to maintain homeostasis.
- **Evening:** As the day progresses, cortisol levels continue to decrease, reaching their lowest point at night. This is important to allow the release of melatonin and prepare the body for sleep.

This pattern repeats every 24 hours, aligning with the body's internal clock, known as the "circadian rhythm." This is why sunlight exposure and circadian rhythm regulation is going to be key when it comes to supporting optimal cortisol production, and we will discuss all this in detail in Step Three: Regulate Your Circadian Rhythm.

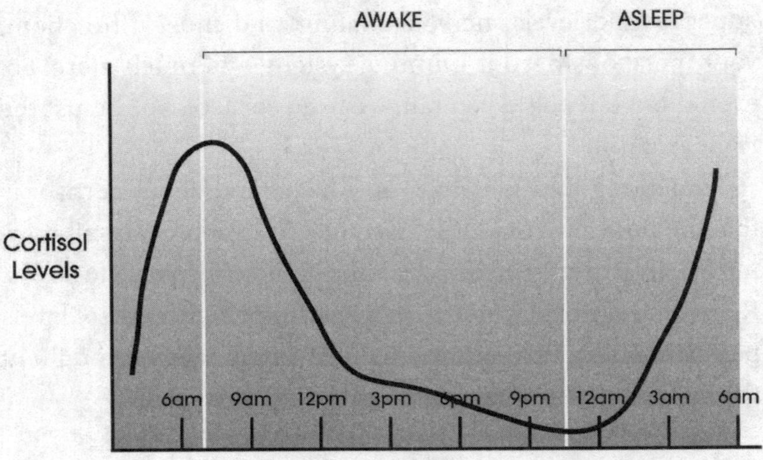

Normal diurnal cortisol rhythm in healthy individuals.

On top of following this daily pattern, cortisol is also released ad hoc in response to threats and stressors. When these stressors are chronic and prolonged, cortisol can become constantly elevated at all times of the day. When this goes on for a while, the body starts to make *adaptations* to protect itself from the damage that could result from prolonged exposure to high levels of this powerful hormone. The body does this by either reducing its sensitivity to cortisol (at a tissue level) or changing the feedback loops that control how much cortisol is produced. The goal is to mitigate the damage of too much cortisol. However, over time, these adaptations might lead to HPA axis dysfunction and disrupt the optimal cortisol production pattern shown above, resulting in various cortisol-related symptoms.[10]

For instance, at first, cortisol might stay elevated all day, making you feel wired, on edge and always rushing from one task to another, and unable to wind down at night. This can progress to adaptations in the HPA axis where production might be higher or lower than normal at specific times, which could make you feel energized before you go to bed when you are supposed to feel sleepy and wake up feeling fatigued and with no energy to start the day. Eventually, the dysregulation in the system might lead to a blunted cortisol response and/or low cortisol levels, making you feel chronically exhausted and unable to adapt to new stressors.

Over time, the dysregulation of the HPA axis has been linked to numerous health issues from symptoms of "burnout," such as emotional exhaustion, physical fatigue, and cognitive problems; to physical health problems, such as heart disease and obesity; and mental health problems, such as depression and anxiety.[11]

- High levels of cortisol have been linked to osteoporosis, hypertension, diabetes, susceptibility to infections, and depression.[12]
- Low cortisol levels, on the other hand, have been linked to CFS, chronic pain, IBS, depression, and difficulty in adapting to both physical and emotional stressors.[13] This is because cortisol plays a critical role in regulating energy, inflammation, and immune responses.

You might be wondering if there is a way to test for stress-related HPA axis dysfunction. The best way to do this is to check the adrenal hormone output of cortisol and the hormone dehydroepiandrosterone (DHEA). DHEA is produced by the adrenal glands, and a balance between cortisol and DHEA is important for overall adrenal health. However, adrenal testing is not something that is routinely checked by clinicians unless there is suspicion of an adrenal disease, such as Addison's disease or Cushing's syndrome (more on these below). Functional doctors and practitioners *do* use adrenal testing, and you can also purchase at-home testing directly from the labs. I have included recommended labs in Appendix A (page 305) if that is something that you might want to explore. However, I recognize that this type of testing can come with a hefty price tag and may not be available worldwide.

In "How the Cortisol Reset Plan Will Help You Thrive," I've therefore included two questionnaires (see pages 47–50) to help you assess your symptoms and determine whether you're experiencing signs of high cortisol, typically associated with the early stages of chronic stress, or low cortisol, often linked to chronic stress that has been endured for a long time and is associated with HPA axis dysfunction. While these questionnaires may not be as accurate as laboratory tests, I've found them beneficial for my clients. I believe they will provide valuable insights for you, too, as knowing whether you have high or low cortisol levels will allow you to access specific tips tailored to your unique needs in the five steps in Part II.

I just want to mention here that stress-related HPA axis dysfunction is not the same as the rare disorders Cushing's disease or Cushing's syndrome (high cortisol) and Addison's disease (low cortisol). Cushing's disease occurs when a tumor on the pituitary gland (known as a pituitary adenoma) makes too much adrenocorticotropic hormone (ACTH). In response, the adrenal glands make too much cortisol. In the case of Cushing's syndrome, excess cortisol can come from outside or inside the body. For example, it can come from using corticosteroid medications or it can come from a pituitary or adrenal tumor causing the body to make too much cortisol. With Addison's disease (also known as "primary adrenal insufficiency"), the adrenal glands are unable to make enough cortisol. Addison's can occur for several reasons, the most frequent being autoimmunity. These diseases are relatively uncommon, but they are both serious conditions that require lifelong management under the care of a doctor.

• • •

By now, I hope you have a solid understanding of what your nervous system does to protect you and keep you alive—how your brain is continuously assessing inputs from your internal and external environment to prepare you to adapt to possible threats, as well as the changes your body makes (the stress response) when it identifies a threat (real or imagined) through allostasis. You also know that these allostatic changes work wonderfully to respond to acute, short-term stressors, but can be damaging when used repeatedly and can lead to allostatic load, which is the burden that stress places on the body and mind and has been linked to negative physical and psychological health problems. When stress does not resolve, the body makes adaptations that can lead to dysregulation in different systems, including the HPA axis.

Thank you for sticking with me! The next chapter is the last deep dive into the science of what is happening in your body, before we get going with the questionnaires and step-by-step plan that will help you reverse the effects of chronic stress.

The Four Types of Stressors

In the middle of difficulty lies opportunity.

—ALBERT EINSTEIN

In the previous chapter, we looked at how stressors can be broadly divided into two groups: perceived (psychological) and physical. Now, let's take it a step further.

In his book *The Role of Stress and the HPA Axis in Chronic Disease Management*, Thomas Guilliams, PhD, explains that, although there are many internal and external threats that affect the HPA axis, most of them can be grouped into four main categories:

1. Perceived stress (emotional and psychological).
2. Circadian disruption.
3. Blood sugar imbalances (glycemic dysregulation).
4. Inflammation (inflammatory signaling).[1]

One of the key goals of the Cortisol Reset Plan is to address and limit each of these categories of stressors so you can stop wasting limited resources dealing with *unnecessary* threats. By reducing unnecessary threats, you will stop overspending and you will be saving up your energy reserves—your "budget." This will allow you to carry out normal day-to-day functions, long-term maintenance and repair functions, and effectively manage the stress response *when needed* to maintain homeostasis, without tipping into maladaptive states. As a result, your cells, organs, and systems will be functioning at their optimal level, ultimately building the resilience needed to thrive and prevent premature ageing and disease.

The goal is not to eliminate *all* stress but to eliminate *unnecessary* stress so you can build your energy reserves and become resilient to stress.

Let's now go deeper into each category.

Perceived Stress

As we've seen, perceived stress is the more "traditional" type of stress that you are most aware of. It's caused by psychological or emotional stressors, which are *anticipatory* and can be real or *imagined*. When thinking about this type of stressor, think worry, anxiety, rumination, fear, panic, hopelessness, or lack of control.

Let's illustrate this: Imagine that you are about to give a presentation in front of 15 colleagues. Your brain is going to assess the situation and compare it with past experiences to predict and assess for a potential threat. Now, this situation might not be a threat if you've never had any issue in the past with public speaking. But if you were laughed at for stuttering while speaking in public as a child, your brain associates similar situations (like giving a presentation now) with the embarrassment and failure you felt then. Your brain will therefore perceive today's presentation as a threat. As a result, your heart rate speeds up, your breathing becomes shallow, you start sweating, and you just want to get out of there as soon as possible (fight or flight). Your mind has triggered the stress response.

But is there a real threat here? There might be, but chances are your colleagues are mature grown-ups who wouldn't laugh at or make fun of you for stuttering while you give a presentation. You can see how, in this case, the activation of the HPA axis and the stress response was "wasteful" since the threat never materialized.

Unfortunately, psychological stressors play a major role (if not the most important role) in causing chronic stress and cortisol dysregulation. This is because humans have highly developed cognitive abilities and are very good at imagining, in incredible detail, potential future scenarios and even better at picturing worst-case scenarios! We do that because our brain hates uncertainty and needs to have some sense of control over what is going to happen, often preparing us for the worst. But our bodies react in the same way to what is happening "in our head" and what is happening in reality.

Perceived stressors are often related to social interactions, but they are also related to financial struggles, work, phobias, information overload, and unresolved trauma. Everybody is going to react differently to these types of stressors because how the brain responds is strongly influenced by different factors, including past experiences (especially during childhood development), trauma, genetic makeup, the balance of neurotransmitters in the brain (the chemical messengers that regulate mood), stress levels, and the degree to which a stressor is perceived as "controllable."[2]

Now, let's focus on how trauma and chronic stress, especially during the critical period of childhood development, can change the "programming" of your nervous system and make you more reactive, hypervigilant, vulnerable, and more susceptible to allostatic load later in life.

TRAUMA AND CHRONIC STRESS

Studies show that chronic stress contributes to changes in brain structures such as the hippocampus, the amygdala, and the prefrontal cortex, which are important for processing memories, regulating emotions, and making decisions.[3] These changes can lead to poor memory, increased fear and anxiety, failure to regulate emotions, and decreased ability to make sound decisions.

But it is not only the brain that might suffer structural changes—vagus nerve function and activity might also be impacted by chronic stress and trauma, with consistent links between lifetime trauma exposures and reduced vagal tone.[4] The vagus nerve plays a crucial role in regulating the parasympathetic nervous system (PNS) by acting as a "brake," slowing the heart rate and helping maintain balance between the sympathetic (fight-or-flight) and parasympathetic (rest-and-digest) systems.

Vagal tone is measured with heart rate variability (HRV), and higher HRV indicates greater flexibility and adaptability. Low HRV is associated with a decreased ability to cope with stressors and has been linked to higher risks of cardiovascular disease, anxiety, depression, IBS, and systemic inflammation.[5]

Here is the silver lining: Both the brain and the vagus nerve have *plasticity*, meaning they can change and adapt in response to new experiences. This means that you are not broken. No matter what your past experiences were, you have the ability to change and become more resilient so you can thrive. You will be learning those skills throughout Part II, but especially in Step Five: Build Psychological Resilience and Well-Being.

No matter how your past experiences, childhood events, or trauma may have shaped your nervous system, you are not broken. You have the power to change, heal, and build resilience.

Circadian Disruption

Circadian disruption is a form of physical stress. It's a real (not imagined) threat to homeostasis. Though it isn't always consciously perceived, it still causes significant disruptions in many systems, contributing to allostatic load.

I cannot stress enough how important the circadian system is in maintaining homeostasis and optimal health. When this system is disrupted, due to irregular sleep patterns, shift work, or lack of sunlight exposure, it can contribute to metabolic disorders, weakened immunity, accelerated ageing, and other health issues.[6]

This is why circadian disruption is considered a major stressor for the body. When circadian disruption is chronic, it can lead to allostatic load and overload as well as HPA axis dysfunction.

There are practical and easy ways to realign your circadian rhythm—and you will learn all about these in Step Three: Regulate Your Circadian Rhythm. Integrating the habits in this step will optimize how your body operates, which will, in turn, boost your capacity and resources (energy), reducing allostatic load.

Blood Sugar Imbalances

Remember from the last chapter how the body is always looking for homeostatic balance? When it comes to blood glucose (blood sugar), your body is always making sure that your levels are not too high or too low, since both can be dangerous.

To understand how closely interrelated the HPA axis and blood sugar regulation are, you need to keep in mind that cortisol is a glucocorticoid. As its name suggests (with "gluco" referring to glucose or sugar), one of cortisol's primary roles is to *increase* blood sugar levels both for everyday metabolic needs and during stress. Why? Because glucose is the primary source of *energy* for most of the body's cells, including the ones in your brain.

The hypothalamus, which is a main player in the stress response, plays a role in the regulation of blood sugar and is very sensitive to changing glucose levels. When blood sugar levels drop too low (known as hypoglycemia), the HPA axis is activated to restore balance, making hypoglycemia a strong trigger for cortisol release.

Low blood sugar can occur if you go too long between meals or fast, but it can also be caused by eating too many carbohydrates or too much sugar at once, which can trigger a spike in insulin followed by a sharp drop in blood glucose. Here's how: When you eat, your body breaks down the food into glucose, which is released into the bloodstream. As blood sugar rises, the pancreas releases insulin to lower it by helping cells absorb glucose for energy or storage.

Eating too much sugar or too many high-carbohydrate foods in a short space of time causes a rapid surge in blood sugar and the release of increased levels of insulin. These insulin surges can cause blood sugar to drop sharply afterward—a phenomenon known as "reactive hypoglycemia." You may be familiar with its symptoms: feeling anxious or grumpy, feeling shaky or light-headed, or having intense cravings. This activates the HPA axis and the stress response.

High glucose → High insulin → Low glucose → Stress response

Over time, consistently high insulin levels can reduce the sensitivity of our cells to insulin (known as insulin resistance). When cells become less responsive, blood sugar levels stay elevated, prompting the body to produce even more insulin to manage the excess glucose. This cycle increases the risk of developing type 2 diabetes and contributes to chronic inflammation.

Interestingly, high blood sugar can also increase cortisol production because elevated glucose levels can cause inflammation. Since one of cortisol's roles is to regulate inflammation, chronic inflammation may prompt the body to produce more cortisol to help manage it.

Now, imagine a typical day of eating that leads to a "blood sugar roller coaster" and the persistent activation of the stress response. You start your morning with a cup of coffee and a piece of toast. Your blood sugar levels increase very quickly and you feel a surge of energy, but it doesn't last long. As your body attempts to manage the sudden spike in glucose, you release a large amount of insulin and you're hit with a crash (low blood sugar levels). This leaves you craving more carb-rich foods, and all of a sudden, the cookies in the office kitchen seem irresistibly tempting.

For your midday meal, you opt for what appears to be a healthy choice: a salad and some fruit. However, the lack of substantial protein and healthy fats leaves you feeling unsatisfied and hungry, contributing to sluggishness and lack of focus in the afternoon. To combat the dreaded afternoon slump, you reach for an energy bar and perhaps another cup of coffee, hoping for a quick fix. While you may experience a brief burst of energy, it's quickly followed by yet another crash, perpetuating the cycle of highs and lows.

As evening approaches, you finally sit down for a proper meal, but you are so hungry that you can't help but eat quickly and possibly more than you really need. You might even feel the need to cap off your meal with something sweet to satisfy cravings, further destabilizing your blood sugar levels and leading to another roller-coaster ride. The resulting spikes and crashes disrupt your sleep, leaving you feeling tired the next morning.

I hope you can see now how both high and low glucose levels are a threat to homeostasis and increase your "stress bucket." But let's take it a step further: Chronic stress increases cortisol levels, and because cortisol is a glucocorticoid, it leads to high blood sugar. This means you can have high blood sugar levels that have nothing to do with what you are eating!

When cortisol is chronically high, blood sugar is also persistently high, leading to elevated insulin levels. This increases your chances of developing metabolic conditions such as obesity, insulin resistance, and diabetes. These conditions are highly inflammatory, and this chronic inflammation further exacerbates stress and disrupts the HPA axis. (Inflammation is another type of stressor that we will cover next.) The interplay between chronic stress, cortisol, metabolic dysfunction, and inflammation creates a vicious cycle, making it difficult to determine which came first: the chicken or the egg.

I know that this might seem a bit complex, but learning to manage your blood sugar through a few simple diet and lifestyle changes, as you will do in Step Two: Balance Your Blood Sugar, will improve your metabolic health, support the proper function of your mitochondria (the tiny powerhouses in your cells) to increase energy levels, decrease inflammation, and help regulate cortisol levels, easing the burden on your adrenal glands.

Inflammation

Inflammation can be acute or it can be chronic. Acute inflammation is the type you may be more familiar with. It's a short-lived response of the immune system to injury or infection. You often associate its symptoms with redness, swelling, heat, and pain. However, not all inflammation is so easy to recognize.

Unlike acute inflammation, chronic inflammation can affect multiple organs throughout the body. It can last for weeks, months, or even years, and it's this sustained inflammatory state that has been linked to many chronic diseases and health conditions.[7] Cortisol is one of the body's most powerful anti-inflammatory hormones and so chronic inflammation increases the demand for cortisol to regulate the immune response, which puts additional strain on the HPA axis. With time, this can contribute to allostatic load and adaptations that blunt the cortisol response or reduce cortisol production, which in turn diminishes its anti-inflammatory effects, contributing to a vicious cycle of inflammation and HPA axis dysfunction.

Chronic inflammation can be caused by many factors:

- **Diet:** Consuming a diet high in processed foods, refined sugars, unhealthy fats, artificial additives, and foods to which you are allergic or sensitive (even if they're deemed "healthy") can exacerbate inflammation.[8] Also, diets low in plant-based foods and healthy fats (such as omega-3 fatty acids) may lack anti-inflammatory nutrients.

- **High blood sugar:** When blood sugar is high, it puts pressure on the mitochondria—your cells' energy producers—to process the excess glucose. This can lead to an overproduction of reactive oxygen species (ROS), which are unstable molecules that, in excess, cause oxidative stress and damage cells. This cellular stress sends danger signals to the immune system, triggering the release of pro-inflammatory cytokines. High blood sugar also causes glucose to stick to proteins and fats in the body—a process called glycation. This creates harmful compounds known as Advanced Glycation End Products (AGEs), which further stimulate inflammation.[9]

- **Poor gut health:** Imbalances in gut microbiota (dysbiosis) where harmful bacteria outnumber beneficial bacteria in the gut, intestinal permeability (leaky gut), and gut infections like parasites or candida can trigger an immune response, leading to inflammation.[10]

- **Autoimmune disorders:** These disorders (such as rheumatoid arthritis, lupus, Hashimoto's, or celiac disease) cause inflammation because the immune system becomes overactive, mistakenly targeting the body's own tissues as if they were foreign invaders.

- **Obesity and metabolic disorders:** When there's too much body fat, particularly visceral fat (which surrounds internal organs), it acts as an active tissue that releases cytokines and adipokines. Cytokines are small proteins that help regulate immune responses, but in excess, they can promote inflammation. Adipokines are also proteins released by fat cells, some of which can have pro-inflammatory effects. When these molecules are released in large amounts, they trigger a state of chronic low-grade inflammation in the body.[11]

- **Sedentary lifestyle:** Lack of regular physical activity or prolonged periods of sitting can lead to inflammation. Exercise has anti-inflammatory effects and helps regulate immune function.

- **Sleep deprivation:** Poor-quality sleep can disrupt immune function and increase inflammation.[12] During sleep, the body repairs tissues and regulates inflammatory responses.

- **Environmental toxins:** Exposure to environmental pollutants, heavy metals, pesticides, and other toxins can trigger inflammation and oxidative stress in the body.[13] Appendix B (page 307) identifies common sources of these toxins and offers simple swaps you can make to significantly reduce your exposure. Be sure to check it out—there's no need for drastic changes. Small, gradual steps can make a big difference over time.

- **Smoking and alcohol consumption:** Both smoking and excessive alcohol consumption have been linked to higher markers of inflammation.[14]

All the strategies you will find in the Cortisol Reset Plan, including minimizing your intake of inflammatory foods, increasing your intake of anti-inflammatory compounds, balancing your blood sugar, strengthening your gut microbiome, repairing your gut lining, and minimizing your exposure to environmental toxins, will help you tackle chronic inflammation so you can decrease allostatic load and improve the functioning of your HPA axis and all the other systems in your body.

• • •

Phew! I know these first two chapters were a lot to take in, but now that you understand how deeply connected your mind and body are, and how chronic stress from both physical and emotional stressors is likely at the root of all your symptoms, the structure of the plan will make much more sense and you'll stop addressing your symptoms in isolation and begin looking at the bigger picture.

Now, let's assess your symptoms and look at how you can reverse the "wear and tear" that chronic stress has caused with the five-step plan.

How the Cortisol Reset Plan Will Help You Thrive

People do not decide their futures, they decide their habits and their habits decide their futures.

—F. M. ALEXANDER

We've seen how many health problems, such as anxiety, depression, metabolic disorders, weight gain, gut issues such as IBS, autoimmune disease, CFS, chronic pain, and many other chronic conditions, are linked to the cumulative burden that chronic stress places on the mind and body. Before we shift our attention to how to reverse the "wear and tear" this chronic stress has caused, let's look at your symptoms and assess whether you have high or low cortisol levels. This will allow you to tailor the plan to your specific needs and track your progress as you implement each step of the plan.

Assess Your Symptoms

In the early stages of chronic stress, we typically experience high cortisol levels, which are linked to symptoms such as feeling wired, insomnia, and weight gain. If stress continues and the allostatic load persists, changes and adaptations in the HPA axis can eventually lead to low cortisol levels. Low cortisol is linked to symptoms such as fatigue, lack of motivation, low blood pressure, and dizziness.

While symptoms can be frustrating, they also serve as valuable messages from your body. Although the strategies you will learn in Part II—for removing the most common sources of stress and improving your capacity and metabolic reserves to become more resilient—will help to improve your symptoms regardless of your cortisol levels, I've included a few targeted recommendations throughout the book to address either high or low cortisol specifically. This can help you fast-track and maximize the benefits and effectiveness of the plan.

Before we get going, I do want to acknowledge that some of you might not be experiencing any symptoms at all or just a few but are still looking to optimize your health and build resilience. Even if you're symptom-free, completing the questionnaires can still be helpful, and know that this book is designed to support you in reaching your optimal health and stress-resilience goals.

In the pages below, you'll find two questionnaires—one for high cortisol symptoms and one for low cortisol symptoms. Each includes several columns: one for you to complete *before* you start the Cortisol Reset Plan and others to complete *after* weeks 2, 4, 6, 8, and 10. Filling out these questionnaires now, before you start the Plan, will help you assess your current symptoms and give you a clear starting point. Repeating them every two weeks will allow you to track your progress over time. Even small improvements can add up—and looking back after a few weeks can reveal just how much has shifted.

Try not to get too caught up in any one score—what matters most is the overall direction. A downward trend in your total score suggests your symptoms are becoming less frequent or intense—which is exactly what we're aiming for.

To make it easy, you can also download a printable version of the questionnaires, along with a cortisol symptom tracker that allows you to chart your progress every two weeks, from my website via the QR code below.

Whether you're completing the questionnaires in the book or using the printable version, the process is the same:

For each symptom, rate how often you experience it using this scale:

0 = Not at all

1 = Occasionally

2 = Frequently

3 = Most of the time

Write the number (0–3) next to each symptom.

Add up all the numbers in the column to get your total score for each questionnaire.

These questionnaires were inspired by those in Dr. Sara Gottfried's *The Hormone Cure* and have been adapted based on my own experience and insights from working with clients and running functional testing over the years.[1]

Questionnaire 1: High cortisol

SYMPTOMS	BEFORE THE CORTISOL RESET PLAN	AFTER WEEK 2	AFTER WEEK 4	AFTER WEEK 6	AFTER WEEK 8	AFTER WEEK 10
I feel anxious or nervous.						
I struggle with calming down before bedtime and often experience a second wind that keeps me up late.						
I wake up in the middle of the night.						
I'm too irritable.						
I crave high-carb foods and sweets.						
I have too many thoughts going on and find it a struggle to focus.						
I have memory lapses.						
I have been putting on weight around my belly.						
I startle easily.						
I lose my temper quickly.						

I feel like I am racing from one activity to the next.						
I use comfort food to help me relax.						
I have skin problems such as eczema or acne.						
My menstrual cycle is irregular.						
My face is puffy; I have a "moon face."						
I am bloated.						
I push myself to do more.						
I feel restless when I am not busy.						
I have high blood sugar.						
I have high blood pressure.						
I have IBS, gastritis, ulcers, or acid reflux.						
Score						

Questionnaire 2: Low cortisol

SYMPTOMS	BEFORE THE CORTISOL RESET PLAN	AFTER WEEK 2	AFTER WEEK 4	AFTER WEEK 6	AFTER WEEK 8	AFTER WEEK 10
I feel completely exhausted.						
It's hard to get excited or motivated to do things.						
I wake up tired, even after a good night's sleep.						
I am sad and melancholic.						
I feel overwhelmed by small things.						
I have muscle weakness.						
My blood pressure is low.						
I feel dizzy or light-headed when I stand up.						
I struggle to recover from illness or wounds.						
I crave salty foods.						
I get sick.						
I feel wiped out after exercising.						

I have chronic pain.						
I have allergies and sensitivities.						
I've experienced a drop in my cognitive agility.						
I can't make decisions.						
I have low blood sugar.						
My appetite is smaller than it used to be.						
I've lost weight or can't put weight on.						
I tend to have a negative outlook in life.						
I have slow digestion, bloating, or gut infections.						
Score						

How to Interpret Your Results

Add up your total scores for each questionnaire.

Compare your scores on the high and low cortisol questionnaires. The higher score shows which pattern—high or low cortisol—is more dominant for you right now. Remember, don't worry too much about the exact number—what matters most is that over time, we want to see your score trending down as your symptoms ease.

Also, you might find that you score high on both questionnaires; this is not uncommon and may suggest that your 24-hour cortisol rhythm is out of sync (see page 27 where we discuss the optimal daily cortisol pattern). In other words, your cortisol may be elevated when it should be low or too low when it should be high. For example, it's common to see high cortisol at night—making it hard to wind down—and low cortisol in the morning, leading to fatigue and difficulty getting out of bed.

I hope these questionnaires have helped you decipher some of the messages and insights your body is sending you. Whatever your score is right now, remember this: You have the ability to rebuild your capacity to cope with stress, recover faster, and reduce or eliminate the symptoms it causes. As your symptoms become less frequent or intense, your scores will gradually go down—a sign that your body is starting to come back into balance.

And just to be clear, the goal isn't to *eliminate* stress entirely, because that's unrealistic. In fact, some level of stress is necessary and beneficial. The goal is to improve your ability to cope and adapt to challenges and quickly reset, restoring balance. I call this *stress resilience*.

Building Stress Resilience

Let's use the analogy of a "stress bucket" to understand stress resilience better.

Your stress levels are the water filling your stress bucket. Each stressor that we explored in "The Four Types of Stressors"—perceived or physical—adds a little more water to the bucket. Over time, if the bucket fills up too much without draining, it will overflow, leading to symptoms and negative health consequences (the allostatic load/overload we saw in "Understanding the Nervous System").

The goal of stress resilience is not to prevent water from entering the bucket, but to improve the capacity of the bucket and the speed at which it drains (how effectively it adapts to each stressor and how quickly it restores balance).

This happens in two ways:

1. **Increase the capacity of the bucket:** To do this, we'll reduce unnecessary stressors that are taking up too much room in your bucket. We'll eliminate physical stressors where possible (like chronic inflammation, sleep disruptions, or blood sugar imbalances) and minimize perceived threats by improving how your brain interprets inputs from the environment. This will stop you wasting resources on unnecessary stress responses. Nervous system regulation through somatic practices and brain rewiring will be key in decreasing perceived stressors.
2. **Increase the resources that help the bucket drain:** Remember that one of the theories of how stress leads to disease is through the energetic cost of redirecting resources from long-term health functions such as repair and maintenance toward short-term survival needs (see page 23 for a reminder on this). The body doesn't have unlimited energy, but you can rebuild and maintain your energy reserves and increase your energy "budget" to make sure you have enough resources for both. This will increase your ability to cope with stressors and boost your resilience to stress-related diseases. We'll achieve this by improving nutrition, optimizing metabolic function, enhancing sleep quality, and incorporating regular exercise.

Stress resilience is about how effectively the body adapts to stressors and how quickly it can reset to balance.

One Habit at a Time

Now, let's talk about *how* we are going to build and maintain stress resilience. In the five-step plan, we are going to make simple and realistic changes to both your diet and your lifestyle. These changes will take a little bit of effort and work at first, but they are going to slowly become automatic through repeated practice (this is the essence of neuroplasticity—your brain's ability to change and adapt in response to new experiences), and they are going to become *habits,* which is key for long-term behavior change.

Habit formation is based on the idea that behaviors become automatic through repeated practice and reinforcement. In his book *The Power of Habit,* Charles Duhigg popularized the "habit loop" model, which explains how habits are created and maintained.[2] This involves three components:

1. The cue (trigger)
2. The routine (behavior)
3. The reward

Forming a new habit starts by initiating a new behavior in response to a specific cue (like a specific time of day, a place or a feeling or emotion). Over time, when we repeatedly do something in response to these cues, our brain links them together, making the behavior automatic. This means that once a habit is formed, we do it without thinking, even if we don't "feel like" doing it.

On the flip side, breaking bad habits is hard because they share the same automatic characteristics as good habits. This doesn't mean it's impossible. It just takes time to swap habits, but with consistent repetition, you can replace old behaviors with new ones.[3] The steps in the Cortisol Reset Plan will help you become more aware of and understand any habits that might not be very helpful and guide you in swapping them for ones that support your long-term healing.

When you are trying to build a new habit, you must get something positive out of it, otherwise you won't continue doing it. This is because when you anticipate a reward (like feeling happy) after a certain behavior, your brain releases dopamine, a neurotransmitter linked to motivation. This positive feedback loop makes it more likely that you'll repeat the behavior in the future.

Let's illustrate this with an example. Say that as soon as you wake up, you always have a cup of coffee. Waking up in the morning is the cue, drinking coffee is the behavior, and that nice boost of energy that coffee gives you is the reward. This is the habit loop that makes this habit stick around.

Now, let's swap this habit loop. We'll keep the same cue—waking up in the morning—but change the behavior to getting outside for a few minutes of natural sunlight. The reward will be boosting your energy levels and improving your mood. This new habit is going to take more time and effort than having a cup of coffee first thing in the morning because you literally need to rewire your brain to link the cue to the new behavior. However, the reward will keep you coming back for more. And the beauty of neuroplasticity is that the more you repeat the new behavior, the stronger the neural connections in your brain will become and, eventually, this new habit will become automatic, no effort required.

The most challenging thing about creating new habits is overcoming the initial resistance from your brain. Your brain prefers the known and familiar over the unknown and will resist any effort from you to change. This is why I cannot emphasize enough how important it is to keep your changes *easy* and manageable. Avoid aiming for huge changes with promises of overnight transformations—they never work and only set you up for failure. Instead, focus on small, achievable changes that compound over time.

"Habit stacking," a term popularized by James Clear and rooted in B. J. Fogg's method of "anchoring," is a great way to make a new habit stick.[4] The idea is to connect a new habit to an existing behavior. For example, after you brush your teeth in the morning (an established habit), you could stack a new habit, such as doing a quick body scan to check in on how you're feeling (the new habit). This technique works because your brain links behaviors to cues and, in this case, the cue is a routine that's already part of your day. Other examples include taking a few deep breaths after drinking water, stretching after a workout, thinking about your intention for the day while you shower, or reading a few pages of a book before bed.

FIVE SIMPLE STEPS TO RESTORE YOUR HEALTH

I have created the Cortisol Reset Plan with this theory of habit formation in mind. I have distilled all my knowledge about creating stress resilience into the simplest and most effective changes that will support long-term healing without overwhelm. To do so, the habits and routines will be introduced gradually, in five different steps, each designed to progress to the next. This ensures that the changes you will be making in each step are manageable and sustainable, and they become habits without having to deal with too much resistance from your brain.

The Cortisol Reset Plan is based on the principle that no matter what your symptoms and health issues are, true healing will happen progressively as you adopt simple and sustainable habits that will compound to big changes over time.

Remember, the ultimate goal of these habits is to rebuild and maintain your stress resilience. As we discussed earlier, this is going to involve reducing unnecessary stressors (physical and perceived) where possible, and to increase your resources (energy) to help your body to quickly and successfully cope and adapt to stressors without triggering maladaptive responses or diverting energy away from essential long-term health functions like repair and maintenance.

The first four steps will focus on decreasing physical stressors as well as boosting your energy reserves. We start with these because the habits in the first four steps are the easiest to implement and will give you almost immediate benefits. The last step will address your perceived stressors. This step is by far the most complex because, as we explored in the previous chapter, the way your brain interprets inputs is strongly influenced by your childhood experiences, trauma, and your current levels of stress. You will likely find more resistance to change here, which is why I have left it for last. By the time you reach this final step, you will be able to tackle it much more successfully once the physical stressors have been taken care of and your energy reserves—your "budget"—are full.

We'll start by reducing your physical stressors and rebuilding your energy reserves, setting you up for success when it's time to tackle perceived psychological and emotional stressors.

Shifting Your Mindset for Lasting Transformation

Before we dive into the Cortisol Reset Plan, I would like to finish this chapter by introducing three mindset shifts that will make the journey a lot more enjoyable and improve your success rate.

CONSISTENCY OVER PERFECTION

Don't let the fear of making mistakes or striving for perfection hold you back. Trying to do too much or to do it perfectly can often leave you paralyzed so you end up not doing anything at all.

Instead, focus on committing to do *something* every day. Some days will feel easy and you will achieve a lot; other days will be harder and you might only do one small thing, and that is enough. Commit to doing at least *one thing*, no matter what. This could be as little as going for a quick walk around the block after lunch or taking a few deep breaths in between meetings. Consistent, incremental progress is what leads to substantial long-term results.

CHANGE HAPPENS ONE SMALL STEP AT A TIME

It's so easy to focus on big changes and overlook the value of small, almost imperceptible daily improvements. But small habits are powerful because they operate on the principle of "compounding"—just like compounding interest in a savings account, incremental progress leads to substantial long-term results. Measure your progress in weeks not days. This is why it's so important to track your progress using the questionnaires once you've started the Cortisol Reset Plan, as it will enable you to see small changes in your symptoms that you otherwise might not have noticed.

YOU ARE YOUR OWN BEST CHEERLEADER

Talk to yourself with compassion and kindness. Be your own ally on this healing journey. Celebrate every win, no matter how small, and recognize how far you've come. At the same time, be honest with yourself about areas in which you can improve and set realistic goals for growth. This mindset will boost your self-confidence and trust in your ability to shape your own future.

> **Remember:** I recommend that you focus on each step for *1 or 2 weeks* before moving on to the next. Your healing journey is not a race, so take the time and trust the process. Let go of the need for immediate results and focus on one day at a time.
>
> Also, avoid comparing yourself to others' healing journeys or getting caught up in too many opinions from social media or podcasts—this can add unnecessary pressure and confusion. Trust that you have a plan that will give you the results you seek if you give it time.

• • •

You are now ready to embark on the first step of the Cortisol Reset Plan and start the journey that will ultimately transform your health.

You've got this!

Part II

The Cortisol Reset Plan

Step One

Eat a Nutrient-Dense Diet

To eat is a necessity, but to eat intelligently is an art.

—FRANÇOIS DE LA ROCHEFOUCAULD

Welcome to the first step of the Cortisol Reset Plan!

You're likely aware that nutrition plays a key role in energy and weight management, but you might be surprised to learn that it is also the foundational building block of stress resilience. The food you eat every single time you have a meal provides the nutrients your body needs to produce and store energy. But food doesn't just provide fuel—it's information; it sends biochemical signals to the body that influence how it functions at a cellular level. Once you think about what food truly does in your body, you'll never be able to look at it in the same way again. It truly is that powerful!

Your meal choices influence things like your hormone levels, inflammation, immune function, metabolism, and more.

More importantly, what you eat influences how your body handles stress as well as how it heals and repairs itself.

In the world of health and wellness, few topics spark as much debate and confusion as nutrition. From epidemiological studies that contradict each other, to sensationalized media stories and the influence of big food companies, figuring out what to eat can feel like a real puzzle. In this step, I want to simplify nutrition so you can make informed decisions to support optimal health.

Demystifying Nutrition

First things first, food is not inherently "good" or "bad," or at least I don't like to vilify food in general, mostly because doing so can lead to an unhealthy relationship with food, eating disorders, and more stress. That said, food does send powerful signals to your body, some that help regulate cortisol and others that throw it off balance. Some foods provide the essential nutrients that support your mitochondria in generating energy efficiently to build stress resilience, while others do the exact opposite. Some help decrease inflammation and oxidative stress, both of which help regulate cortisol, while others increase them, making it harder for your body to recover from stress.

This is why addressing food first in the Cortisol Reset Plan is so important. You eat multiple times a day, every day, meaning you have plenty of opportunities to reduce dietary stressors that contribute to cortisol dysregulation (such as foods that increase inflammation), while simultaneously improving your metabolic and energetic reserves to enhance stress resilience.

Also, nutrition isn't just about the foods themselves. We also have to take into account that we are all different, and factors like genetics, metabolism, lifestyle, and environment can all influence how your body responds to what you eat.

Let's illustrate this with an example. Is dairy "healthy"? Well, that's a bit of a complex question! Dairy products like milk, yogurt, and cheese can be highly nutritious. However, the "healthiness" of dairy can vary depending on several factors. First, quality matters. Milk from pasture-raised cows may contain higher levels of beneficial nutrients compared to milk from grain-fed cows. Similarly, the processing methods used, such as homogenization, can also impact the nutritional content. And, more importantly, individuality is crucial. Some people may have lactose intolerance or dairy allergies, which can make consuming dairy products problematic and detrimental to their health.

So here's my approach to nutrition: First, evidence is important and that is why I rely on peer-reviewed research, including systematic reviews, meta-analyses, randomized controlled trials (RCTs), and large observational studies. These provide a solid foundation for my recommendations, but I also consider how humans have evolved over millennia to eat certain foods, prioritizing those in my advice. And lastly, I take into account individuality: If a certain food doesn't agree with you, it doesn't matter how healthy the most reputable study says it is!

The nutrition recommendations outlined in this first step are based on two principles:

1. First, we'll focus on consuming nutrient-dense foods that provide the essential macronutrients and micronutrients necessary for optimal health. When your body receives the right nutrients, maintaining a healthy weight becomes easier, as your metabolism is optimized and cravings are naturally reduced. I will also introduce some specific nu-

trients and food sources that have been shown to support the HPA axis and the stress response.

2. Second, we'll address inflammation through dietary changes. Chronic inflammation is a physical stressor and is linked to weight gain. A diet high in processed foods, refined sugars, unhealthy fats, artificial additives, and even foods to which you may have a sensitivity (even if they're deemed "healthy") can exacerbate inflammation.

Ultimately, navigating the complexities of nutrition requires cutting through the noise and finding what works for *you*.

I hope this chapter will provide you with all the info you need to navigate the world of nutrition with confidence and ensure that every choice you make is a step toward the strong body and calm mind we're striving for.

Before we dive into the weeds of nutrition, let's pause to discuss a simple and free habit that can transform how your body digests and absorbs nutrients.

Be More Present

In many cultures, mealtimes are a chance to *slow down* and connect with the people we care about. Although modern life can make these moments harder to come by, we can still bring that sense of presence and connection to our meals, even in small ways.

This might mean sitting down instead of eating on the go, or simply taking a deep breath before your first bite and slowing down a little. These simple habits support better digestion and give you space to truly enjoy your food.

Now, let's explore why *how* you eat matters just as much as *what* you eat. Being "here" in the present moment when you are eating your meals is something that you probably don't do very often, but it's something that you can cultivate and make part of your daily routine. It involves paying close attention to the act of eating—looking at your food, smelling it, tasting it, noticing the textures in your mouth—and ultimately, it's about *slowing down* and enjoying each bite.

Let's try a quick exercise that will help you grasp what this means. You may be familiar with this if you have ever completed a mindfulness course. I did this many years ago and I found it so transformative that I have been teaching it to my clients and course students ever since!

Find something small to eat, like a raisin, and take just one. Hold it in your hand and look at it closely. What does it look like? What color is it? What is its texture? Now, put it in your mouth and move it around with your tongue. Notice its texture: Is it wrinkled or smooth? Is it plump or dry? Next, chew it slowly: Is it sticky on your teeth? What does it taste like? Is it sweet? Finally, swallow it and observe how you feel afterward. Did you enjoy the experience?

I'm not suggesting that you eat every meal with such meticulous attention, but I encourage you to reflect on how you felt during this exercise, because it captures the essence of what being here in the present moment really means. You probably found that, while you were eating that raisin, time slowed down and you fully immersed yourself in the experience. This shift in attention away from past and future worries and toward the present moment promotes relaxation and activates the PNS, which, as we saw in "Understanding the Nervous System," is also called "rest and digest," leading to better digestion and improved gastrointestinal function.[1]

Now, compare the way you ate that raisin with your usual approach to meals. I bet you often find yourself doing a few things at the same time: ensuring your kids are eating, working while you eat, watching a show, or scrolling through your phone. These activities often keep your SNS and stress response activated.

In this state, your body is putting digestion on hold because it needs to deal with more urgent needs. This often disrupts the regular muscle contractions along the digestive tract and reduces the secretion of essential digestive enzymes. For example, have you ever read an urgent message in the middle of your meal or dealt with your kids arguing at the table? I bet you ate quickly to get the meal over and done with as soon as possible, but perhaps felt bloated and uncomfortable afterward.

While we don't have direct control over our digestion, we do have the ability to activate our PNS before meals and *indirectly* influence our digestion. This is because the PNS, primarily through the vagus nerve, plays a key role in regulating the release of saliva and gastric and pancreatic juices to break down food, as well as promoting the movement of food through the gut and supporting nutrient absorption.[2]

Another benefit of eating mindfully is improving interoception—your ability to sense internal bodily signals. This helps you recognize when you're truly full, reducing the chance of overeating.

Here are four strategies that can help you become more present when you eat:

1. **Sit down and minimize distractions:** Make mealtimes intentional by sitting down and creating a calm eating environment. Turn off the TV and set aside your phone.

2. **Cultivate gratitude:** Before diving into your meal, take a moment to express gratitude for the nourishment before you. This can take the form of a formal prayer or a simple acknowledgment of the efforts of those involved in bringing the food to your table.
3. **Take a deep breath:** Before your first bite, take a deep breath with a long exhale.
4. **Slow down:** Slow the pace of your meal by thoroughly chewing each bite. Allow your saliva to mix with the food. This helps break down food mechanically and chemically, making digestion easier. Eating slowly also gives your digestive system time to activate enzymes and release hormones that prepare your gut for efficient digestion and nutrient absorption.

To form the habit of being more present when you eat, concentrate on these four key practices during *just one* meal per day. This way you'll attach the behavior of being present to that specific meal, allowing you to gradually build the habit over time by repeating it. For example, practice these four strategies each time you have lunch (this is the cue) and, with repetition, it will become automatic. Then you can do the same with breakfast and dinner.

> **Remember the habit loop we met in the previous chapter: cue (meal) → behavior (being present) → reward (better digestion).**

By paying close attention to the present moment when you are eating, you can boost digestion, improve your relationship with food, and become more attuned to your body's signals.

Now that you have learned a few key habits to improve *how* you eat, let's focus on *what* to eat to decrease your stress and optimize your health.

Choose the Best Fuel for Your Body

Growing up in a part of Spain famous for its love of food and high-quality produce, I was lucky to be surrounded by a diverse and wholesome diet from a very early age. Our table was always filled with lots of plant-based foods (fruits, vegetables, whole grains, nuts, and beans) along with plenty of olive oil (and I mean plenty!), raw cheeses, yogurt, meat, fish, and other minimally processed and locally grown ingredients.

The dietary recommendations in this step are deeply influenced by my Spanish heritage but are also grounded in science, since the Mediterranean diet has been extensively studied for decades for its ability to reduce the risk of chronic diseases, especially cardiovascular disease, metabolic conditions, and cancer prevention, due to its anti-inflammatory and antioxidant properties.[3]

This means we will be focusing on a colorful variety of fresh, unprocessed foods that will provide your body with macronutrients (protein, fats, and carbohydrates), micronutrients (vitamins and minerals), and beneficial compounds like antioxidants, polyphenols, prebiotics, and probiotics. All these will improve mitochondrial health and energy production, reduce inflammation, and support gut health. (Don't worry—we'll be looking at exactly what each of these is in just a moment.)

I will also discuss how to minimize the consumption of inflammatory foods. However, as I've mentioned, I want to move away from a culture of demonizing foods—these foods are not "evil" and won't harm you if you eat them every once in a while, but they do cause issues in the long term and need to be limited as much as possible.

My goal is to make this way of eating enjoyable and satisfying while naturally supporting your optimal weight. Once you begin to experience its benefits, you won't want to turn back! If you want to get started straight away, you'll find plenty of recipes for breakfast, lunch, and dinner in Part III (page 261).

Let's now dive into this way of eating. And to make it easy to follow, I've grouped all foods into three main macronutrients: protein, carbohydrates, and fats. It's important to include foods from all these three categories in each meal because each plays a unique role in supporting your body's overall health and energy. Every food contains at least one of these macronutrients, though many foods include a combination of all three, with one typically being dominant. For example, an apple is primarily carbohydrates, olive oil is almost entirely fat, and milk contains a mix of protein, carbohydrates, and fat.

Beyond macronutrients, whole foods contain essential micronutrients and other beneficial compounds. As we go along, I'll discuss these in more detail and show you how they fit into this way of eating.

PROTEIN

The word "protein" comes from the Greek word *proteios*, meaning "primary." This should already give you a clue about how important eating enough protein is! Think of protein as the raw material needed to repair cells, build muscle, and create essential compounds like hormones and neurotransmitters.

Protein is essential for growing and repairing tissues in the body, including muscles, joints, skin, hair, and nails. It also plays a crucial role in supporting the immune system, detoxification processes, and digestive health. Additionally, protein is important for mental health, as it helps your body make neurotransmitters, which are chemical messengers that help regulate mood, contributing to overall mental well-being.

Proteins are made up of 20 amino acids, which are like building blocks. Some amino acids are essential, meaning the body can't make them and must get them from food. The rest are nonessential and can be made by the body.

Protein-rich foods can come from both animal and plant sources. While both contain essential amino acids, there are some differences. Animal proteins generally provide all essential amino acids in the right proportions and are more "bioavailable," meaning they are easier to absorb and use by your body. Plant proteins, while still valuable, often lack one or more essential amino acids and can be less bioavailable because they are not as easy to absorb and use. This doesn't mean that plant proteins are ineffective, but they may require more variety and pairing of different plant-based protein sources to help ensure you get all the essential amino acids your body needs.

The other benefit of animal proteins is that they contain certain important micronutrients that are challenging to get from plant-based sources, including vitamin B12, vitamin A (retinol), heme iron (the form of iron that is most easily absorbed by the body and is mostly found in meat and seafood), omega-3 fatty acids (particularly eicosapentaenoic acid [EPA] and docosahexaenoic acid [DHA]), zinc, and creatine.

So, overall, a combination of animal- and plant-based proteins is best. If you are vegetarian, it's possible to get enough high-quality protein if you also eat dairy and eggs. This can be more challenging on a strictly vegan diet, although not impossible! If you're vegan, you may need to rely on supplements to prevent getting deficiencies.

You are probably wondering how much protein to aim for each day. Unfortunately, as with most things in nutrition, there's no simple answer. Your optimal protein intake depends on your gender, age, weight, and physical activity. I have given you a few guidelines below, but know that you might have to do a little bit of experimentation until you find your sweet spot.

You'll know you're getting the right amount of protein when you feel satisfied after meals, have steady energy, and can build and maintain muscle with exercise. If you're always hungry, struggle to gain muscle, or feel sluggish, you might need more. On the other hand, too much protein can sometimes lead to digestive issues like constipation, especially if you're not eating enough fiber-rich plant foods. I often see this with people who focus so much on animal protein that they forget to include enough plant-based foods. Too much protein can also contribute to weight gain if it leads to an overall calorie surplus, so just keep that in mind—more isn't always better. The key is finding the right balance for your body.

The Recommended Dietary Allowance (RDA) for protein to prevent deficiency for adults is 0.8 grams of protein per kilogram of body weight, or 0.36 grams per pound.[4] However, recent research suggests that higher protein intakes—typically ranging from 1.2 to 1.6 grams per kilogram of body weight per day, or 0.54 to 0.73 grams per pound—could provide added health advantages, especially in addressing age-related muscle loss, supporting weight management, and improving athletic performance.[5]

When you calculate how much protein you are currently eating, you might find that you're hitting your protein target. However, people often tend to eat protein unevenly throughout the day: They skimp on it in the morning and load up in the evening. For optimal absorption and use, it's better to spread your protein intake evenly throughout the day. Research suggests that evenly splitting your protein intake is key to supporting muscle repair and growth.[6]

On top of that, protein is very satiating; it keeps you full, which helps control appetite, prevents overeating, and supports better weight management. By spreading your protein intake evenly across meals, you can better manage your hunger and stabilize your blood sugar levels, ensuring that you have sustained energy and mental focus throughout the day.

For example, if you weigh 145 pounds, first convert your weight to kilograms by dividing by 2.2 (145 ÷ 2.2 ≈ 66 kg). Based on the guideline of 1.2 to 1.6 grams per kilogram of body weight, your optimal protein intake would be roughly 79 to 106 grams per day. To spread this evenly across three meals, aim for roughly 26 to 35 grams of protein per meal. Here's what that could look like in a day:

- Breakfast (≈29 grams protein): Greek yogurt (1 cup = ~20 grams protein) with chia seeds (1 teaspoon = 1 gram protein), hemp seeds (1 tablespoon = 3 grams protein), and a handful of almonds (1 ounce = 5 grams protein), topped with berries.

- Lunch (≈32 grams protein): Grilled chicken breast (3 ounces = 27 grams) with quinoa (½ cup cooked = 4 grams), roasted vegetables, and a tahini dressing (1 tablespoon tahini = 1 gram).

- Dinner (≈31 grams protein): Baked salmon (4.25 ounces = 26 grams) with mashed sweet potato and a leafy green salad with pumpkin seeds (1 tablespoon = 5 grams).

Below is a list of excellent sources of protein. I have calculated their approximate protein using the USDA Food Database.[7] Note the foods are cooked when applicable (meat, fish, and beans, for example). Protein content can vary slightly depending on factors like brand, preparation method, and fat content.

Using a kitchen scale initially can be helpful to develop a clear visual of portion sizes and how they look in real life.

Animal Protein Chart

ANIMAL PROTEIN SOURCE	SERVING	APPROXIMATE PROTEIN CONTENT
Chicken breast	3 oz.	27 g
Beef tenderloin	3 oz.	25 g
Cottage cheese	1 cup	25 g
Turkey breast	3 oz.	25 g
Sardines	3.5 oz.	25 g
Prawns/shrimp	3.5 oz.	24 g
Beef liver	3 oz.	23 g
Bison	3 oz.	23 g
Lamb	3 oz.	23 g
Snapper	3.5 oz.	23 g
Tuna	3.5 oz.	23 g
Chicken legs/thighs	3 oz.	22 g
Pork	3 oz.	22 g
Salmon	3.5 oz.	22 g
Cod	3.5 oz.	20 g
Crab	3.5 oz.	20 g
Greek yogurt	1 cup	20 g
Eggs	2 large	12 g
Milk	1 cup	8 g
Halloumi cheese	1 oz.	6 g
Beef isolate protein powder	1 oz. (1 scoop)	25 g
Whey protein powder	1 oz. (1 scoop)	25 g

Plant Protein Chart

PLANT PROTEIN SOURCE	SERVING	APPROXIMATE PROTEIN CONTENT
Tempeh	3.5 oz.	19 g
Tofu (firm)	3.5 oz.	17 g
Hemp seeds	1 oz.	9 g
Lentils	½ cup	9 g
Black beans	½ cup	8 g
Chickpeas	½ cup	8 g
Edamame (soybeans)	1 oz.	8 g
Kidney beans	½ cup	8 g
Pumpkin seeds	1 oz.	8 g
Adzuki beans	½ cup	7 g
Lima beans	½ cup	7 g
Peanuts	1 oz.	7 g
Almonds	1 oz.	6 g
Chia seeds	1 oz.	5 g
Green peas	½ cup	5 g
Sunflower seeds	1 oz.	5 g
Amaranth	½ cup	4 g
Quinoa	½ cup	4 g
Sorghum	⅓ cup	4 g
Rice protein powder	1 oz. (1 scoop)	24 g
Pea protein powder	1 oz. (1 scoop)	22 g

When choosing animal proteins, prioritize products that offer the highest quality and are within your budget:

- If possible, opt for grass-fed when it comes to beef and other grass-eating livestock. This means the animals have been grazing on open pasture so they have been eating grass (not grains) all their lives. The meat of grass-fed animals is richer in beneficial nutrients compared to that of grain-fed animals.

- If grass-fed options are unavailable, choose organic meats. Organic meats come from animals raised without antibiotics or hormones and are fed an organic diet free from genetically modified organisms (GMOs).
- When choosing chicken and eggs, opt for pasture-raised when possible. Pasture-raised chickens are allowed to roam freely outdoors and forage on grass and bugs. This leads to eggs and chicken that are higher in nutrients.
- For fish and seafood, choose wild-caught options over farmed whenever possible. Wild-caught fish are sourced from natural marine environments and tend to be higher in beneficial nutrients like omega-3 fatty acids compared to farmed options. Look for labels indicating wild-caught fish and prioritize sustainable options certified by organizations like the Marine Stewardship Council (MSC).
- Consider purchasing fish that is low in mercury and other contaminants, such as salmon, sardines, flounder, trout, tilapia, cod, or sole. Avoid larger fish like shark, swordfish, and marlin, which tend to accumulate higher levels of mercury.
- When it comes to dairy products, opt for organic and grass-fed options that come from cows that have been raised without antibiotics or hormones and allowed to graze on natural pasture. Unhomogenized options (such as milk with the cream at the top) are less processed and better for your health.

- When choosing a protein powder, always check the label for unwanted additives, artificial flavors, or sweeteners. A good-quality protein powder can be a great way to boost your protein intake, but I suggest using them as a supplement not a replacement for whole foods. Aim to get most of your protein from natural food sources and use protein powder for an extra boost when needed. For example, you might add a tablespoon or two to your yogurt or oatmeal in the morning to help reach your protein goal.

- Though it has fallen out of favor in recent years, I also encourage you to incorporate liver into your diet. This often overlooked cut is not only cheap, it also provides a lot of nutrients (it's one of the richest sources of micronutrients like vitamins A and B12, iron, folate, and copper). For an easy way to add liver to your diet, try mixing finely chopped or ground liver into your ground beef when making Bolognese sauce or meatballs. A good proportion is about 1 part liver to 4 parts ground beef, so the flavor isn't too overwhelming. You can adjust the ratio to suit your taste, but this is a great starting point.

The second habit to introduce (after mindful eating) is to ensure you're including a source of protein in each meal. You can refer to the list above and choose one or two protein sources that help you reach your target. Alternatively, you can check out the recipes in Part III (page 261), where I've included options with at least 25 grams of protein per serving. For example, you could try the Overnight Quinoa and Raspberry Yogurt Bowl (page 268) for breakfast, the Tempeh and Avocado Salad with Tahini Dressing (page 274) for lunch, and the Roasted Herb Chicken and Veggies (page 279) for dinner.

CARBOHYDRATES

Carbohydrates are often misunderstood and blamed for weight gain. But carbs aren't evil!

If protein is good at building your body, carbs are good at giving your body energy. In fact, they are the body's preferred source of energy.

When carbohydrates are available, the body will prioritize using them for fuel before turning to fats or proteins. They are vital for brain function, support thyroid health, aid in metabolism, and are essential for proper muscle function. Additionally, carbohydrates are often an excellent source of dietary fiber, promoting digestive health and maintaining a healthy gut microbiome. Beyond their physical benefits, carbohydrates also influence serotonin levels, contributing to mood stability and overall well-being.

When we consume carbohydrates, they are broken down into glucose, which is consumed by cells to create energy. Excess glucose is either stored in the liver or muscles (in the form of glycogen) and released as needed, or in adipose tissue (fat cells) as fat.

Glucose is so vital for our health that if we don't get enough from food or when glycogen stores are depleted (which happens after periods of fasting or after intense exercise), our body can produce it from non-carbohydrate sources, primarily through a process called "gluconeogenesis." (Hormones like cortisol, glucagon, and adrenaline [epinephrine] stimulate gluconeogenesis, and we will explore more about this in Step Two, including why low glucose levels trigger the stress response.) When carbs are very low for a prolonged period, the body shifts to burning fat instead of glucose as its main source of energy. This shift is known as ketosis, a metabolic adaptation that helps maintain energy levels when glucose is scarce, allowing the body to function without carbs. You might be familiar with the ketogenic or keto diet, which is designed to encourage this metabolic shift to promote fat loss by heavily restricting carbs. While the keto diet can be effective for short-term weight loss, the reality is that maintaining ketosis requires reducing carbohydrate intake to a point where meeting your daily fiber and nutrient requirements becomes very challenging. The long-term effects of ketosis remain unclear and, for many people, this restrictive diet can lead to nutrient deficiencies, digestive issues like constipation, and fatigue.

So, while carbohydrates might not be biologically necessary, they are a quick source of energy, and some of them have a lot of micronutrients and fiber. And, of course, let's not forget, they are delicious! Think fruit and vegetables, grains, dairy, and honey.

Luckily, we don't need to eliminate carbs from our diet, but it is also true that plenty of carbohydrate-rich foods aren't very good for us. This is why it's important to think about the *quality* of the carbohydrates you consume each day so you are making the best choices for building stress resilience.

There are three main categories of carbs:[8]

1. **Sugar:** Sugar is the simplest form of carbohydrate. It occurs naturally in some foods, including fruit and dairy. Types of sugar include fruit sugar (fructose), table sugar

(sucrose), and milk sugar (lactose). Added sugars can also be found in many foods, such as cookies, cake, ice cream, sugary drinks, and candy.

2. **Starch:** Starches are complex carbohydrates made up of long chains of sugar molecules. They take longer to digest compared to sugars and provide a more sustained release of energy. Starches are found in foods like grains (wheat, rice, oats), legumes (beans, lentils, chickpeas), and starchy vegetables (potatoes, pumpkin, squash).
3. **Fiber:** Dietary fibers are nondigestible carbohydrates found in plant-based foods. They pass through the digestive system largely intact and provide various health benefits, including promoting digestive health, supporting weight management, and helping control blood sugar levels. Fiber-rich foods include whole grains, fruits, vegetables, nuts, seeds, and legumes.

Fiber and starch are complex carbs, while sugar is a simple carb. Complex carbohydrates are digested more slowly, releasing glucose into the bloodstream gradually. In contrast, simple carbohydrates are digested quickly, causing blood sugar to spike faster and higher—and then drop.

The nutrient quality of a food depends on how much of each of these components it contains. Fruit, for example, contains both simple and complex carbohydrates. The main carbohydrate in fruit is sugar (fructose), which is a simple carbohydrate. However, fruits also contain fiber, which is a complex carbohydrate. The combination of these two components makes fruits a source of both simple and complex carbohydrates. Fruit juices, on the other hand, are a source of simple but not complex carbohydrates because the fiber has been removed.

The Cortisol Reset Plan emphasizes the complex carbs found in vegetables, whole fruits, whole grains, and legumes. These sources provide a steady release of energy and are rich in essential nutrients and fiber. It's these whole foods that you should prioritize in your diet.

When it comes to simple carbs, we will be limiting some sources, such as table sugar, white bread, white flour, pastries, fruit juice, sweets, and sweetened beverages. While dried fruit, honey, molasses, and maple syrup are simple carbs with more nutrients, they can still spike blood sugar levels, so they should be used sparingly. If you currently have a lot of these simple sugars in your diet, please don't worry. This change doesn't need to happen overnight. It's about slowly phasing out the less nutritious options and replacing them with better alternatives. This process can be gradual and, as always, I want you to take it one step at a time.

Take Petra, for example, one of my clients. She used to love having a KitKat after lunch, and it became a comforting part of her daily routine. Rather than simply eliminating this habit and feeling deprived, Petra swapped her KitKat for a piece of dark chocolate and a date. After a few days, she gradually replaced the date with a handful of almonds. Her new routine of having a piece of dark chocolate and a few almonds not only gave her similar feelings of comfort and satisfaction, but she also noticed that she started feeling better in the afternoon. After a few days, her cravings for sweets began to fade. Just like Petra, you can start by making small swaps in your diet, one step at a time.

Does this mean you should never eat sugar again? Not at all. Life wouldn't be fun without a sweet treat here and there! You will find, though, that as you transition to a nutrient-dense diet, cravings for cookies, cakes, doughnuts, potato chips, and similar treats start to fade. This is because your body begins to feel more satisfied and nourished by the foods it truly needs, helping reduce the urge for less nutritious options.

Don't stress over the occasional treat

Remember, no food is inherently "good" or "bad." The goal is to crowd out less nutritious choices with foods that will support your health in the long term. What matters most is the food you *consistently* choose every day. So, if you want to eat a cupcake because it's your birthday, go ahead and enjoy every bite!

To minimize the risk of blood sugar spikes when you eat carbohydrates, you'll learn to balance your intake by pairing it with adequate protein and healthy fats, which help stabilize blood sugar levels and promote satiety. I'll also share some strategies to prevent carb-induced blood sugar spikes in the next step of the plan: Balance Your Blood Sugar.

Below are two lists: one of carbs to prioritize and another of carbs to limit or avoid. In the list of carbs to prioritize, you'll notice some vegetables that you might not typically associate with "carbs." For example, leafy greens are high in fiber and packed with micronutrients. While they are low in net carbs, they provide the fiber and essential vitamins and minerals, and other beneficial compounds that will optimize your health.

Carbohydrates to prioritize

TYPE OF CARBS	FOOD SOURCES	
Fruits *These are rich in simple sugars (fructose) and fiber. They are also very high in micronutrients and other beneficial compounds.* Portion per day: 1–2 servings. For example: 1 apple, pear, or orange (~1 serving) 2 small apricots or plums (~1 serving) ½ cup fresh berries (~1 serving)	• apple • apricot • blackberries • blueberries • cantaloupe melon • cherries • cranberries • grapes • guava • honeydew melon • kiwi • lemon	• lime • mango • orange • papaya • peach • pear • pineapple • plum • pomegranate • raspberries • rhubarb • strawberries • watermelon
High-starch vegetables *These are rich in starches and fiber. They are high in micronutrients and other beneficial compounds.* Portion per day: 1–2 servings. For example: ½ cup cooked sweet potato, squash, or mashed potatoes (~1 serving) 1 medium baked potato or parsnip (~1 serving)	• acorn squash • beetroot • butternut squash • carrot • corn on the cob • delicata squash • kabocha squash	• parsnip • potato • pumpkin • spaghetti squash • swede (rutabaga) • sweet potato • turnip
Low-starch vegetables *These are rich in fiber and have high amounts of micronutrients such as vitamins, minerals, plus other compounds such as phytonutrients.* Portion per day: Unlimited servings (at least 4–5 servings encouraged). For example: 1 cup raw leafy greens (spinach, kale, etc.) (~1 serving) ½ cup cooked non-leafy vegetables like broccoli or cauliflower (~1 serving)	• asparagus • arugula • beetroot greens • bok choy • broccoli • Brussels sprouts • cabbage (green, red) • cauliflower • celery • collard greens • cucumber	• dandelion greens • eggplant • endive • garlic • green beans • kale • lamb's lettuce (mâche) • leek • lettuce (romaine, iceberg, butterhead)

	• mushrooms (shiitake, portobello) • mustard greens • onion • peppers (bell pepper, chile pepper) • radicchio • radishes • sea vegetables (nori, kombu)	• shallot • sorrel • spinach • spring onions • sprouts (alfalfa, broccoli) • Swiss chard • tomato • watercress
Grains *These are rich in starches and fiber.* Portion per day: 1 serving. For example: ½ cup cooked quinoa, oats, or brown rice (~1 serving) 1 slice or 1.5 oz. whole-grain bread (~1 serving)	• amaranth • barley • brown rice • buckwheat • bulgur • corn • cornmeal • farro • Kamut • millet • oats (including	rolled and steel-cut) • rye • sorghum • teff • quinoa • wheat (whole wheat, durum, spelt) • wild rice
Legumes/beans *These are rich in starches and fiber. They are high in micronutrients and other beneficial compounds.* Portion per week: 2–3 servings per week. For example: ½ cup cooked lentils, chickpeas, or black beans (~1 serving) Add to soups, salads, or side dishes three times per week.	• adzuki beans • black beans • black-eyed peas • butter beans • cannellini beans • chickpeas (garbanzo beans) • fava beans (broad beans)	• kidney beans • lentils • lima beans • mung beans • navy beans • pinto beans • split peas (green or yellow)
Dried fruit (in moderation) *Dried fruits are rich in simple sugars and fiber, and they provide micronutrients. However, due to their high sugar content, they should be consumed in moderation.*	• dates • dried apricots • dried blueberries • dried cranberries	• dried figs • dried mango • dried raisins

Natural sweeteners (in moderation; use sparingly) *These are rich in simple sugars and provide some micronutrients but should be consumed in moderation due to their high sugar content.*	• coconut sugar • date syrup • honey • maple syrup • molasses

Carbohydrates to limit or avoid

TYPE OF CARBS	FOOD SOURCES
Refined sugars	• corn syrup • high-fructose corn syrup (HFCS) • table sugar
Sweets and pastries	• cakes • candy/lollipops • cookies • doughnuts • milk chocolate bars or chocolate bars that have less than 70 percent cacao • pastries
Drinks	• chocolate milk • fruit juices • soda • sweetened iced tea
Processed grain products and starches	• bagels (whole-grain or sprouted versions are better alternatives) • crackers (whole-grain or sprouted versions are better alternatives) • chips • highly processed white bread (sourdough, whole-grain, or sprouted bread are more nutritious options) • sweetened breakfast cereals • white pasta (okay in moderation but whole-grain or legume-based pasta is a better option) • white rice (okay in moderation; cooking and cooling overnight in the fridge increases resistant starch [a type of fiber with many health benefits] and lowers the glycemic index of rice, making it a bit less impactful on blood sugar levels than freshly cooked rice)

I know this section might feel like a lot, but don't worry—I'm guiding you through this, step by step. The third habit we're going to focus on is making sure you add a source of complex carbs to each of your meals. Just like we did with protein, take a look at the carb options I've recommended and aim for 1 serving at each meal. You can pick fruit, vegetables, grains, or legumes (you can find the serving size on the left side of the chart). For example, if you've chosen Greek yogurt for breakfast as your protein source, add a serving of fruit on top, like ½ cup of blueberries. For lunch, if you've picked grilled chicken, pair it with a serving of sweet potato and arugula. For dinner, if tofu is your protein, try adding chopped broccoli and mushrooms in a stir-fry and serve with quinoa. If you prefer, you can also pick any of the recipes in Part III (page 261).

If you're used to having simple sugars as a regular part of your diet, try using the approach we did with Petra—rather than depriving yourself, focus on swapping out less beneficial sources of carbs for healthier alternatives. For example, if you often reach for fizzy drinks or fruit juice, try sparkling water with a splash of lemon juice instead. Or, if you enjoy a sweet snack in the afternoon, swap store-bought cookies or a sugary granola bar for a handful of mixed nuts and a couple of dried apricots. These small changes will help you crowd out less nutritious options while still satisfying your cravings with better choices.

FAT

Here is another macronutrient, along with carbs, that has been the subject of a lot of debate and contradictory opinions for years, but the truth is that a certain amount of fat in our diet is not only delicious, but it is also beneficial and necessary for our health.[9]

Fat provides your body with energy, and it plays a role in cellular function, neurological health, the absorption of fat-soluble vitamins (A, D, E, and K) and hormonal balance, influencing everything from mood regulation to hormone synthesis. By incorporating some fats into your diet, you can support metabolic function, reduce inflammation, stabilize blood sugar levels, and support sustainable weight management by providing satiety. But, of course, not all fats are created equal, and some are better than others.

There are four main types of fats. Ideally, we should prioritize polyunsaturated and monounsaturated fats, consume saturated fats in moderation, and avoid trans fats:

1. **Polyunsaturated fats (PUFAs):** Polyunsaturated (along with monounsaturated) fats are often referred to as "healthy fats," and they tend to be liquid at room temperature. They are considered essential fats because the body cannot produce them, so they must be obtained from the diet. There are two main types: omega-3 and omega-6 fatty acids, both of which play crucial roles in overall health. Omega-3s, particularly EPA and DHA (found in fatty fish), are especially beneficial for brain function, heart health, and reducing inflammation.
2. **Monounsaturated fats (MUFAs):** Monounsaturated fats are also referred to as "healthy fats" and remain liquid at room temperature. They are found in foods like extra-virgin olive oil, avocados, nuts, and seeds. MUFAs are

known for their heart-protective benefits, as they help improve cholesterol levels, reduce inflammation, and lower oxidative stress. Studies have linked extra-virgin olive oil, in particular, to better cardiovascular health, making it a key component of the Mediterranean diet.[10]

3. **Saturated fats:** Saturated fats are typically solid at room temperature and are found primarily in meat and dairy products, and some plant sources like coconuts. They have been traditionally associated with negative health effects like increasing total cholesterol and the risk of heart disease, but recent research has provided mixed findings on their impact. A review of 15 RCTs showed that reducing saturated fat had little to no effect on overall mortality, cardiovascular deaths, or key health markers like cholesterol, blood pressure, and BMI. While there were small reductions in weight and cholesterol, the impact was minimal.[11] The findings are still debated, and more research is probably needed, but in my opinion, consuming *small* amounts of saturated fats sourced from nutrient-dense foods in their natural state, like grass-fed beef, butter or ghee (clarified butter) from grass-fed cows, virgin coconut oil, or full-fat dairy products from grass-fed animals, is okay.
4. **Trans fats:** Trans fats are the worst type of fat and should be avoided because their consumption has been linked to inflammation and heart disease.[12] This type of fat is made by "hydrogenating" oils to make them solid and more shelf stable. Fortunately, trans fats have been banned in many countries, but they might still be found in small amounts in certain foods, particularly in margarine, pro-

cessed baked goods, and other packaged products that use hydrogenated oils.

Note that many foods contain a combination of two or more types of fat. But there is often a predominant one. For example, walnuts contain a mix of polyunsaturated fats (omega-3), monounsaturated fats (oleic acid), and small amounts of saturated fat.

Navigating fats can feel a bit confusing, but don't worry—you just need to keep a few simple guidelines in mind:

1. Avoid trans fats.
2. Limit saturated fats (and choose quality sources when you do eat them).
3. Prioritize MUFAs and PUFAs from the right sources.

To help you incorporate these guidelines into your diet more easily, I've created a list of healthy fats to include (with the best food sources) and a list of fats to avoid.

When it comes to portions, be mindful that fats are calorie-dense (providing 9 calories per gram, compared to 4 calories per gram for protein and carbs), so it's important to keep portions reasonable (which can be tricky with nuts, as it's easy to overdo it!). A typical serving size for healthy fats could be a handful of nuts (1 ounce), 1 tablespoon of olive oil, half an avocado, or 4.25–5.0 ounces of fatty or oily fish.

Fats to enjoy

TYPE OF FAT	FOOD SOURCES
Polyunsaturated fats	• **Fatty or oily fish**, including salmon, mackerel, trout, sardines, and herring, are excellent sources of omega-3 fatty acids, notably EPA and DHA. These omega-3 fatty acids play vital roles in reducing inflammation, supporting brain health, and aiding stress management. EPA and DHA are also essential components of brain cell membranes and are integral to neurotransmitter function, influencing mood regulation and cognitive performance.[13] • **Flaxseeds** are a rich, plant-based source of alpha-linolenic acid (ALA), a type of omega-3 fatty acid. While ALA is not as potent as EPA and DHA, found in fatty fish, it can still provide benefits. • **Sunflower and pumpkin seeds** are high in omega-6 fatty acids and one of the best sources of vitamin E. • **Walnuts** are an excellent source of omega-3 fatty acids, particularly ALA, which can help reduce inflammation and support heart health. They are also rich in antioxidants like vitamin E, which can protect cells from oxidative stress. *Note: Vegetable and seed oils or "cooking oils" (such as soybean, sunflower, cottonseed, and grapeseed) are high in polyunsaturated fats but should be consumed in moderation (see below for more details).*
Monounsaturated fats	• **Almonds, macadamia nuts, hazelnuts, pistachios, and cashews** are good sources of monounsaturated fats. They also provide protein, fiber, and nutrients like vitamin E and magnesium. • **Avocados and avocado oil** have been linked to improving cardiovascular health, supporting weight loss, enhancing cognitive function, and promoting gut health.[14] • **Olive oil (extra-virgin) and olives** are rich in antioxidants and oleic acid, and have been linked to improved heart health, reduced inflammation, and lowered risk of chronic diseases. • **Peanuts** are an excellent source of monounsaturated fats and plant-based protein. • **Sesame seeds** are high in monounsaturated fats and minerals like selenium, calcium, and magnesium.

Saturated fats (in moderation)	• **Butter and ghee** derived from the milk of grass-fed cows are rich in vitamins A, D, E, and K2, as well as omega-3 fatty acids and conjugated linoleic acid (CLA). Ghee is heat stable, making it suitable for cooking at high temperatures. • **Cocoa butter** is the natural fat extracted from cocoa beans and it is rich in saturated fats, particularly stearic acid. It is commonly used in chocolate making and baking, and has antioxidant properties. • **Full-fat dairy products**, such as milk, cheese, and yogurt, from grass-fed animals contain higher levels of omega-3 fatty acids, CLA, and vitamins than conventional dairy products from grain-fed animals. • **Grass-fed beef** contains saturated fat but also higher levels of omega-3 fatty acids and CLA compared to grain-fed beef. These nutrients have been associated with various health benefits. • **Virgin coconut oil** is high in lauric acid, a type of saturated fat with antimicrobial properties. Additionally, coconut oil is heat stable, making it suitable for cooking at high temperatures.

Trans fats should be avoided, and polyunsaturated fats from refined vegetable and seed oils (cooking oils) should be limited, even though they are polyunsaturated fats.

Refined vegetable and seed oils have been under debate for the last few years. They might be problematic for a couple of reasons; first, by the way they are processed. This involves high temperatures and solvents that can generate harmful compounds such as free radicals and oxidized fats. Additionally, these oils tend to be high in omega-6 fatty acids, and diets disproportionately high in omega-6 fats and deficient in omega-3s have been linked to inflammation.[15] For this reason, I recommend choosing better food sources of polyunsaturated fats as mentioned above.

Fats to avoid/limit

TYPE OF FAT	FOOD SOURCES	
Trans fats **Avoid**	Trans fats are banned or heavily regulated in many countries, making them easier to avoid. However, it's still important to check the ingredient labels of packaged foods. Even if a product claims to be free of trans fats, if "partially hydrogenated oils" are listed on the label, it still contains some amount of trans fats.	
Refined vegetable and seed oils **Limit**	• canola oil • corn oil • cottonseed oil • grapeseed oil • rapeseed oil	• safflower oil • soybean oil • sunflower oil • vegetable oil (a blend of various refined oils)

Consider the smoke point of fats

When selecting a fat for cooking, it's crucial to consider its smoke point: the temperature at which it starts to break down, leading to the formation of harmful compounds such as free radicals and other oxidation by-products.

For high-heat cooking (above 400°F), use oils with high smoke points, such as avocado oil or ghee (clarified butter). These fats can withstand high temperatures without breaking down or producing harmful compounds.

Extra-virgin olive oil has a lower smoke point, making it better suited for low- to medium-heat cooking (up to 325–400°F) or for use cold to drizzle over vegetables or in dressings.

Oils like flaxseed, almond, or unrefined sesame oil are extremely sensitive to heat, light, and air, which can cause them to oxidize and become rancid when exposed to high temperatures. It's best to avoid cooking with these oils and to store them in a cool place. Use them cold, such as for drizzling over dishes or as ingredients in dressings, to preserve their nutritional integrity.

Let's just take a moment to consider how you can incorporate the right types of fats into your diet—this is the fourth habit to focus on:

- Polyunsaturated fats (especially omega-3) should be included regularly. Aim to have fatty fish like salmon, mackerel, or sardines once or twice a week. If you're not a fan of fish, consider supplementing with fish or cod liver oil. Other good sources of polyunsaturated fats include flaxseeds, chia seeds, walnuts, and hemp seeds.
- Monounsaturated fats should also be part of your diet. These can be included by cooking with avocado oil, using 1 tablespoon of extra-virgin olive oil in your salad, or adding half an avocado to your toast. A small handful of almonds, pistachios, or hazelnuts are also a great option.
- Saturated fats should make up a *small* portion of your diet from healthy sources such as grass-fed beef or full-fat dairy from grass-fed cows.
- Swap refined cooking oils for avocado oil (for high-heat cooking) or extra-virgin olive oil (for medium- or low-heat cooking).

Now that you have a good understanding of the three macronutrients, aim to include a source of each in every meal. For example, when preparing dinner, start with a protein source like chicken breast, add plenty of low-starch vegetables like broccoli or kale, and select either a high-starch veggie like sweet potato, grains like wild rice, or legumes like lentils. Finish the meal with a healthy fat, such as a drizzle of extra-virgin olive oil. Keep in mind that some foods, like salmon or steak, provide both protein and fat, so you might not need to add extra fat.

Meal formula: protein + carbohydrates (low starch + high starch *or* grain *or* legumes) + fat

Use the table below to create a meal plan for the next week. Don't worry—I've included plenty of recipes in Part III (page 261) to help you get familiar with creating balanced meals like this.

	BREAKFAST	LUNCH	DINNER
MONDAY			
TUESDAY			
WEDNESDAY			
THURSDAY			
FRIDAY			
SATURDAY			
SUNDAY			

Remember: Your brain doesn't like change and will always prefer sticking to what is familiar. To overcome this, you need to make changes as small, easy, and convenient as possible. Take it slow, enjoy the journey, and trust that small but consistent efforts will compound into real transformations over time.

Use Your Diet to Decrease Inflammation

A lot of the changes you've already made—such as eating enough high-quality protein, prioritizing complex carbs, and switching to healthier fats—will have gone some way to reducing inflammation, but let's now look in detail at how to further enhance gut health and decrease inflammation.

As you learned in "Understanding the Nervous System," inflammation is a common physical source of stress that contributes to allostatic load, cortisol dysregulation, and HPA axis dysfunction. We saw that the most common causes of chronic inflammation include eating inflammatory foods, high blood sugar, poor gut health, obesity, sleep deprivation, alcohol consumption, and more.

Decreasing inflammatory foods and improving gut health are "low-hanging fruits" that provide the most bang for your buck when it comes to reducing inflammation. That's exactly what you'll learn to do here through simple dietary changes. These include eliminating reactive foods from your diet, incorporating prebiotic, probiotic, and polyphenol-rich foods to improve your gut ecosystem (microbiome), and supporting the gut barrier with targeted nutrients. I've also included a few gut-healing recipes in Part III (see page 261).

LIMIT INFLAMMATORY FOODS

There are several foods or ingredients in foods that have been shown to trigger inflammation, so try to stay clear or limit your intake of these foods as much as possible to help decrease inflammation.

Processed meats

Processed meats have been cured with salt and synthetic nitrates to boost their flavor and/or extend their shelf life. Some of the most common examples include cold meats, bacon, hot dogs, pepperoni, salami, and deli meats. Observational studies have linked a high intake of processed meat to a higher risk of cardiovascular disease, and a systematic review and meta-analysis found significant associations between processed meat consumption and the incidence of various cancer types.[16] The World Health Organization (WHO) has classified processed meats as being carcinogenic to humans.[17] If you do choose to eat processed meats occasionally, look for options that are free of synthetic nitrates or nitrites, which are typically replaced with natural preservatives like salt or celery powder (which contains naturally occurring nitrates). Of course, as we discussed earlier, it's best to eat unprocessed, good-quality meat from healthy, well-raised animals.

Highly processed foods

Processed foods are often loaded with artificial chemicals and compounds that don't naturally occur in food, like artificial sweeteners, preservatives, artificial flavors, emulsifiers, and chemicals leaching from food packaging. Research has linked a diet high in ultra-processed foods (UPFs) to increased inflammation, partly because of their effects on gut health and microbiome balance.[18] Here are some easy swaps that will help you decrease your exposure to UPFs:

- Swap sugary snacks like candy or packaged cookies for fresh fruit, a date stuffed with a teaspoon of peanut butter, or a piece of dark chocolate (more than 70 percent cacao).

- Swap sodas and energy drinks for sparkling water with a splash of lemon juice or pomegranate juice.
- Swap packaged breakfast cereals for oatmeal made with rolled oats served with fresh fruits, nuts, and seeds.
- Swap store-bought salad dressings for a simple homemade version by mixing together 3 tablespoons of extra-virgin olive oil, 1 tablespoon of vinegar, 1 teaspoon of Dijon mustard, freshly ground black pepper, and a pinch of salt.
- Swap a packet of potato chips for homemade stovetop popcorn.

Refined carbohydrates

Foods made with refined grains, such as white bread, pasta, cookies, and crackers, often undergo extensive processing, stripping them of beneficial nutrients and fiber. They can cause spikes in blood sugar levels, leading to inflammation. Instead, choose whole grains like quinoa, wild rice, oats, farro, and barley, along with whole-wheat bread, whole-wheat or legume pasta, and whole-grain or seed-based crackers, which contain fiber that helps to stabilize blood sugar and reduce inflammation.

Added sugars

Excessive consumption of sugary foods and beverages, including sweets, pastries, fizzy drinks, and fruit juices, can promote inflammation. Try to limit your intake of added sugars and satisfy your sweet tooth with fresh fruits or a small portion of dark chocolate instead.

Trans fats

We discussed trans fats on page 87. They are commonly found in processed and fried foods, margarine, and certain packaged snacks. These fats are notorious for causing inflammation in the body. To avoid trans fats, steer clear of foods with "hydrogenated" or "partially hydrogenated" oils in the ingredients list. Since 2018, artificial trans fats have been banned in the US following the FDA's ruling on partially hydrogenated oils (PHOs).[19] However, small amounts (less than 0.5 grams per serving) can still appear in some packaged foods and may be labelled as 0 grams on nutrition panels. To catch hidden trans fats, always check the ingredients list for "partially hydrogenated oils."

Refined vegetable oils

Refined vegetable oils like canola, sunflower, cottonseed, soybean, corn, safflower, grapeseed, and rice bran are high in omega-6 fatty acids, which, when consumed in excess, can disrupt the balance of omega-6 with omega-3 fatty acids in the body. While omega-6 fatty acids are essential for health, getting too much of them, especially when they are consumed in a disproportionate ratio to omega-3 fatty acids, could promote inflammation.

To avoid using these oils, swap them for the alternatives outlined on page 92. Also, keep in mind that refined vegetable oils are commonly used in restaurant kitchens because of their neutral flavor, high smoke point, and low cost. While you can't have control over what's used when dining out, you can control how many times you eat out every week. Dining out occasionally is perfectly fine, but aim to make it a treat rather than a daily habit, focusing on home-cooked meals whenever possible.

Artificial sweeteners

Artificial sweeteners like aspartame and saccharin have been linked to inflammation by potentially disrupting the balance of gut bacteria and triggering inflammatory pathways.[20] While more research is needed, evidence suggests that we should consume artificial sweeteners in moderation.[21] Instead, swap them for natural sweeteners like raw honey, maple syrup, stevia, or monk fruit.

Alcohol

Excessive alcohol consumption can disrupt gut health, leading to inflammation and increased permeability of the intestinal lining (known as leaky gut). Studies also show that drinking large amounts of alcohol can increase certain inflammatory markers.[22] Consider limiting alcohol by choosing alternatives like kombucha or mocktails made with sparkling water, herbs, and fresh fruit. Another great option, especially when you're out socializing, is to switch to 0 percent alcohol drinks, such as nonalcoholic beers, wines, or sparkling beverages. These provide the look and familiar taste of alcohol without the negative side effects.

Are there any inflammatory foods you can think about excluding from your diet this week? You don't have to eliminate them all, but think about what you tend to eat frequently and make one simple swap.

REMOVE FOOD TRIGGERS

There are foods that aren't inherently "inflammatory" and may even be considered "healthy," but they can still trigger inflammation in some people, which is often referred to as food sensitivity or intolerance.

Before diving into the most common triggers, it's important to understand the key differences between an intolerance and an allergy. In the case of a food allergy, the immune system produces a specific kind of antibody (known as "immunoglobulin E") when exposed to a particular food. The reaction is typically immediate and can range from mild symptoms, like hives, rashes or itching, to life-threatening reactions (anaphylaxis), where the throat swells and breathing becomes difficult, requiring urgent medical attention, typically with the use of an adrenaline (epinephrine) injection (EpiPen).

Food intolerances, on the other hand, are different and can be harder to identify because the symptoms are not as severe and reactions don't necessarily occur immediately after eating the food. Symptoms of food intolerance can vary widely and may include digestive issues, headaches, or skin problems.

In this book, you won't find blanket recommendations to eliminate foods such as gluten-containing foods or dairy. That's because I don't believe most people need to cut out these foods from their diet, and removing major food groups should always be done under the guidance of a healthcare professional.

I will, however, share what the most common triggers are so you can pay attention to how you feel after you eat those foods. If you suspect a food sensitivity, I encourage you to talk with your doctor or dietitian. They can help you safely explore an elimination diet to identify potential triggers.

Gluten-containing foods

Found in wheat, barley, and rye, gluten is one of the most common triggers of inflammation, particularly in individuals with either celiac disease or gluten sensitivity.

Celiac disease is an autoimmune disorder characterized by serious systemic inflammation and damage to the small intestine triggered by the consumption of gluten. This damage can lead to poor absorption of nutrients through the gut, resulting in various nutritional deficiencies. Additionally, people with celiac disease are at an increased risk of developing other autoimmune conditions.[23] Symptoms include pain, diarrhea, bloating, fatigue, nutrient deficiencies, weight loss, and neurological symptoms.

However, gluten can be problematic for people without celiac disease. This is called non-celiac gluten sensitivity (NCGS) and its symptoms can include things like bloating, gut pain, fatigue, headaches, joint pain, and sometimes neurological symptoms. It's not autoimmune in nature but can still lead to chronic inflammation.

Gluten can be found in a wide range of grains and grain-based products, including wheat, barley, rye, spelt, Kamut, triticale, semolina, farro, durum, bulgur, couscous, malt, wheat bran, wheat germ, and products derived from these grains, such as bread, pasta, cereal, baked goods, beer, and many processed foods.

Dairy

Dairy is a highly nutritious food that has nourished humans since we domesticated ruminants more than 10,000 years ago, but not everyone can tolerate it.

"Milk intolerance" is a broad term that includes various adverse reactions to milk or dairy products, including both lactose intolerance and nonallergic adverse reactions to components in milk. While lactose intolerance specifically refers to difficulty digesting lactose due to enzyme deficiency, milk intolerance may include intolerance to other components in milk, such as proteins like casein or whey. Symptoms of lactose intolerance are primarily gut-related, including bloating, gas, diarrhea, and cramps. On the other hand, symptoms of milk intolerance can be broader and may include digestive issues, skin problems, respiratory symptoms, or other adverse reactions.

Nightshades

Nightshade vegetables, like tomatoes, peppers, potatoes, and eggplants, contain compounds that may exacerbate inflammation in some people, particularly those with autoimmune conditions like arthritis or Hashimoto's. For some people, consuming nightshades can trigger symptoms such as joint pain, skin flare-ups, or gut issues.

High-histamine foods

Some foods, especially those that are aged or fermented, naturally contain high levels of histamines or can trigger the release of histamines in the body.

People who are sensitive to histamines might experience a range of symptoms when they eat foods that are naturally high in histamines, including skin rashes, digestive issues, abdominal pain, bloating, diarrhea, nasal congestion, headaches, anxiety, or fatigue.

High-histamine foods include aged cheeses, fermented foods, processed meats, dried fruit, alcoholic beverages (especially red wine and beer), certain fruits and vegetables (for example, citrus, tomatoes, avocados, and spinach), and leftover foods, as histamine levels increase the longer food is stored in the fridge (freezing leftovers can help prevent histamine buildup, making them a better option for those who are sensitive).

Other potential food triggers you might want to keep in mind are soy, corn, eggs, sulphites, and yeast. While this list is not exhaustive, it includes the "common suspects" often associated with food intolerances.

Did any of these symptoms resonate with you? If so, speak to your doctor or dietitian about your options.

ADD GUT-HEALING FOODS

In addition to avoiding inflammatory foods and those you may be sensitive to, I'd like you to consider incorporating specific foods that will support a healthy gut microbiome and strengthen the gut lining. This can help reduce gut inflammation and promote overall digestive health.

Think of your gut microbiome as a living ecosystem in your gut with a diverse community of microorganisms, including bacteria, fungi, viruses, and other microbes. Some are beneficial, while others are not, but the diversity and balance between them is what truly matters.

More and more studies are emerging showing that the microbiome plays a huge role in most aspects of our health, including digestion, immune function, metabolism, and mood regulation. In fact, having a diverse microbiome (a wide variety of different types of microorganisms living in the gut) has been shown to offer several benefits:

- **Nutrient absorption and energy management:** A diverse microbiome plays a key role in breaking down and absorbing nutrients from food. It also helps regulate how the body uses and stores energy from the food we eat, influencing how efficiently the body processes food and manages energy.[24]

- **Stronger immune system:** The gut microbiome plays a crucial role in regulating the immune system.[25] A diverse microbiome helps maintain a balanced immune response, and a balanced *and* diverse microbiome helps regulate inflammation in the gut and throughout the body.

- **Weight management:** Studies have shown that a diverse microbiome may be associated with a healthier body weight.[26] Imbalances in gut bacteria have been linked to obesity and metabolic disorders.

- **Improved brain function and mental health:** A diverse microbiome is associated with a lower risk of mood disorders like depression and anxiety. Microbes in the gut produce neurotransmitters like serotonin and dopamine, which play a role in mood regulation. Research suggests that a diverse microbiome may also benefit cognitive function and brain health.[27]

We have the power to influence the health of our gut microbiome, and achieving this relies on consuming a diverse diet rich in nutrients that support the growth and diversity of these microorganisms. This is what you have learned to do so far, by eating a nutrient-dense diet that includes carbohydrates, proteins, fats, vitamins and minerals, and other beneficial compounds found in a wide array of foods to nourish different species of gut bacteria and foster microbial diversity.

On top of that, if you want to give your gut an extra boost, consider incorporating the following foods into your diet:

Probiotic foods

Probiotic foods are fermented foods that contain live beneficial bacteria. When we eat them, these live bacteria colonize the gut, contributing to a more diverse gut microbiome. Consuming probiotic-rich foods can help maintain a balanced gut microbiome, improve digestion, boost immunity, and support your mood. *Lactobacillus*, commonly found in fermented food, has been linked to stress management and potential prevention of depression and anxiety![28] Some examples of probiotic foods are yogurt, kefir, sauerkraut, kimchi, miso, tempeh, and kombucha. Always buy these fermented foods from the refrigerated section of the supermarket, as they will have the most probiotic bacteria. You can also make your own at home for a fraction of the cost—I've included a super-easy recipe for Homemade Sauerkraut in Part III (see page 296).

Prebiotic foods

Prebiotic foods are rich in dietary fibers that "feed" the beneficial bacteria in the gut, promoting their growth. These fibers are not digested by the body but instead reach the colon, where they are fermented by gut bacteria.

When prebiotics are fermented by gut microorganisms, they produce short-chain fatty acids (SCFAs) such as butyrate, acetate, and propionate. These SCFAs are linked to several benefits, including less inflammation, better digestive health, better mineral absorption, improved blood sugar regulation, and strengthened immune support.[29]

Here are the best sources of prebiotics:

- Fruits: bananas (especially green), apples, pears, berries, and citrus fruits

- Grains: rye, oats, quinoa, and buckwheat

- Legumes: chickpeas, lentils, kidney beans, black beans, and navy beans

- Seeds: flaxseeds, and chia seeds

- Vegetables: chicory root, dandelion greens, garlic, onions, leeks, asparagus, artichokes, potatoes (especially when cooked and cooled), fennel bulbs, and green peas

I also want to mention again here that cooking and cooling starchy foods like potatoes and rice can increase their resistant starch content. Resistant starch is a type of prebiotic that has plenty of benefits, including better blood sugar regulation, better insulin sensitivity, and increased post-meal satiety.[30] You should just cook it as usual and then refrigerate for a few hours or overnight. (Safety tip: Rice can be problematic if not stored or handled correctly. After cooking, refrigerate it within 1 hour and consume within 2 days. If left out for longer than 1 hour, discard it. Improperly stored rice can harbor harmful bacteria like *Bacillus cereus*.)

Polyphenol-rich foods

Polyphenols are plant compounds that have gained significant attention in recent decades for their significant health-promoting benefits, including their antioxidant properties, ability to reduce inflammation, fight bacteria, and protect brain health.

Interestingly, many polyphenols have low bioavailability, meaning they are not absorbed and instead reach the colon, where they interact with gut microorganisms (much like prebiotics). There is growing evidence that they promote the growth of beneficial bacteria such as *Bifidobacterium* and *Lactobacillus*, while reducing harmful bacteria. This shift in bacterial composition is linked to an increase in SCFAs, which help reduce inflammation.[31]

Below is a list of polyphenol-rich food sources that have been shown to improve the composition of gut bacteria:

- berries (blueberries, raspberries, blackberries, goji berries, elderberries)
- cacao and dark chocolate
- coffee and tea (black, green, oolong)
- ginger (see more benefits of ginger for gut health below)
- grapes
- nuts and seeds
- oranges
- pomegranates
- tart cherries

Bone broth

Simple to prepare and so nourishing for the gut, bone broth is one of the oldest and most budget-friendly home remedies. It is done by simmering bones from animals such as chicken, beef, lamb, or fish in water over a long period, typically 12–24 hours.

A good-quality bone broth is full of collagen, gelatin, and essential amino acids like glycine, proline, and glutamine, which are all important for supporting the integrity of the gut lining. These nutrients support the growth and regeneration of gut epithelial cells, helping in the healing and sealing of a leaky gut.

I've included two recipes for bone broth (beef and chicken) in the Gut-Healing Recipes section in Part III (see pages 294 and 295). It can be enjoyed on its own or added to soups, stews, and smoothies, or even be used to cook rice or quinoa.

Ginger

Ginger has a long history of use in traditional medicine for supporting digestive health. It contains compounds such as gingerol, shogaol, and paradol, which have anti-inflammatory properties. It has also traditionally been used to soothe digestive discomfort, including nausea, indigestion, bloating, and gas. You can simply add fresh or powdered ginger to your cooking, or you can make ginger water using the recipe provided in Part III (page 297) and sip it between meals.

Which gut-healing foods could you look to incorporate this week?

CONSIDER GUT-HEALING SUPPLEMENTS

By adopting the type of diet we have discussed so far—a diverse diet rich in unprocessed foods—and by limiting inflammatory triggers and incorporating pro- and prebiotic foods, polyphenol-rich foods, bone broth, and ginger, you're already providing your gut with everything it needs to thrive!

However, it is true that supplements, while not necessary, can accelerate gut healing, especially for those who have symptoms of gut problems already. Below, I've introduced a range of supplements known to enhance digestion, improve nutrient absorption, balance the gut microbiome, and support repair of the gut lining. Please always check with your doctor before starting a new supplement to make sure they are appropriate for you.

Digestive enzymes

Digestive enzymes are essential for breaking down the food you eat into smaller components so that your body can absorb nutrients more efficiently. These enzymes help with the digestion of proteins, fats, carbohydrates, and fibers, ensuring that your body gets the maximum nutritional benefit from food.

You naturally produce digestive enzymes, but you can take a supplement to improve digestion, especially if you suffer from bloating or slow digestion. When choosing a digestive enzyme supplement, look for one that contains a broad spectrum of enzymes, including amylase for carbohydrates, protease for proteins, lipase for fats, and lactase for lactose (especially for those with lactose intolerance). Some supplements may also include betaine HCl, which can further support digestion, especially in those with low stomach acid.

Herbal bitters

Herbal bitters are plants or plant extracts that have a bitter taste and are known to stimulate the vagus nerve and the digestive system. Herbal bitters stimulate the production of digestive juices, including stomach acid and bile, which aids in the digestion and absorption of nutrients. They also promote peristalsis, the movement of food through the digestive tract. Bitter herbs include gentian root, dandelion root, artichoke leaf, burdock root, orange peel, yellow dock, and angelica root. Note that herbal bitters should be avoided when pregnant.

Probiotics

Certain strains of probiotics, such as *Lactobacillus* and *Bifidobacterium*, are known to restore the normal balance of gut flora and enhance the integrity of the gut barrier. Research has also linked these probiotic strains to improvements in mood and reductions in symptoms of anxiety and depression. For example, *Bifidobacterium longum* has been shown to reduce perceived stress,[32] while *Lactobacillus plantarum* has been shown to improve stress and anxiety symptoms.[33]

Another beneficial option is *Saccharomyces boulardii*, a probiotic yeast that supports gut health by inhibiting the growth of harmful bacteria and restoring microbial balance. *S. boulardii* might increase secretory immunoglobulin A (sIgA) levels, strengthening the junctions between intestinal cells and reducing the permeability of the gut barrier.[34]

If you want to add some gut-healing supplements to your diet, speak to your doctor about which might be most appropriate for you.

Add Nutrients That Support Your Stress Response

Now that you've learned how to adjust your diet to enhance gut health and reduce inflammation, addressing some of the most common physical stressors, let's talk about specific nutrients (and food sources) that are not only nutritious but have also been linked to being able to support the HPA axis and help to regulate the release of cortisol and the overall stress response.

In Part I, you learned how the stress response is resource-intensive: The body requires a lot of energy to sustain it, and it also increases your need for certain vitamins and minerals. Your body burns through these nutrients more quickly under stress, which is why it's so important to replenish them through your diet to maintain resilience. Replenishing nutrients is crucial whether you have symptoms of high or low cortisol. However, if you scored higher on the low cortisol questionnaire on page 49, be especially mindful. In my experience, those with low cortisol are more likely to have nutrient deficiencies, and they might want to consider supplements alongside food to help fill in the gaps.

Let's look at what the key nutrients are.

VITAMIN C

Vitamin C supports adrenal health and function, ensuring the efficient production of cortisol. It is also a potent antioxidant that scavenges free radicals, reducing oxidative damage to cells and tissues. Additionally, it supports the synthesis of neurotransmitters, which control mood and stress response. In some studies, people reported that vitamin C lowered their anxiety levels.[35] Consuming 300–500 milligrams of vitamin C per day may be beneficial for supporting adrenal function and managing stress.

Vitamin C is found in many fruits and vegetables; below are some of the best sources for this powerhouse.

SOURCE OF VITAMIN C	APPROXIMATE CONTENT PER 3.5 OZ
Guava	228 mg
Bell pepper (red)	127 mg
Kale	93 mg
Kiwi	93 mg
Broccoli	89 mg
Brussels sprouts	85 mg
Papaya	60 mg
Strawberries	59 mg
Orange	53 mg
Pineapple	47 mg

If you're considering using supplements to increase your vitamin C intake, I recommend opting for a whole-food vitamin C supplement derived from real food sources. Typically, these supplements contain ingredients like camu camu powder or acerola powder, which are berries naturally rich in vitamin C that have been finely powdered for easy consumption.

MAGNESIUM

Magnesium is involved in more than 300 biochemical reactions in the body and plays a crucial role in regulating the nervous system, muscle function, and neurotransmitter release.[36] Stress not only depletes magnesium, but magnesium deficiency itself can increase mood issues such as anxiety and depression.[37] Magnesium can help increase stress resilience by improving sleep quality and also by improving fatigue, since magnesium boosts energy by supporting cellular energy production. It can also improve metabolic function by enhancing glucose metabolism and insulin sensitivity.[38] The RDA for magnesium, set by the National Institutes of Health (NIH), is approximately 400–420 milligrams per day for men and 310–320 milligrams per day for women, with higher recommendations during pregnancy and lactation.[39] Below are some key sources of magnesium.

SOURCE OF MAGNESIUM	APPROXIMATE CONTENT PER SERVING
Pumpkin seeds (1 oz.)	168 mg
Chia seeds (1 oz.)	111 mg
Spinach (½ cup, cooked)	78 mg
Almonds (1 oz.)	76 mg
Cashews (1 oz.)	74 mg
Dark chocolate (70–85 percent cacao, 1 oz.)	64 mg
Black beans (½ cup, cooked)	60 mg
Avocado (1 medium)	58 mg
Edamame (½ cup, cooked)	50 mg
Yogurt (plain, 1 cup)	47 mg
Lentils (½ cup, cooked)	36 mg
Banana (1 medium)	32 mg

Considering all of the important roles that magnesium plays in the body and the fact that it is quickly depleted under chronic stress, sometimes it's a good idea to consider taking magnesium supplements on top of eating magnesium-rich foods. However, it's best to check with your doctor to ensure you're getting the right dose and type for your needs.

Magnesium supplements are available in different forms:

- **Magnesium citrate:** This is highly absorbable and is often used to promote bowel regularity and relieve constipation. It may cause loose stools or diarrhea, especially in higher doses.

- **Magnesium glycinate:** This form is well absorbed and less likely to cause digestive issues because it has minimal laxative effects.

- **Magnesium L-threonate:** This has shown promise in crossing the blood-brain barrier and supporting cognitive function. It may improve memory and cognitive performance. However, limited research is available on its long-term effects.

- **Magnesium malate:** Magnesium malate is often used to support energy production and alleviate symptoms of fatigue. It combines magnesium with malic acid, which may improve absorption and support the process your body uses to make energy (known as ATP synthesis). This type is best taken in the morning.

- **Magnesium chloride:** This is typically used topically in the form of magnesium oil or flakes for transdermal absorption. It may cause skin irritation.

- **Magnesium taurate:** Magnesium taurate combines magnesium with the amino acid taurine and is often promoted for cardiovascular health. It may support heart function and regulate blood pressure.

OMEGA-3 FATTY ACIDS

Omega-3 fatty acids have anti-inflammatory properties that help regulate the body's immune response and reduce chronic inflammation. Omega-3 fatty acids also play a role in regulating neurotransmitter function and inflammation in the brain, which can influence mood and mental health. Studies have shown that omega-3 supplementation may reduce symptoms of depression, anxiety, and other mood disorders.[40]

Oily or fatty fish is the best food source for omega-3 fatty acids. It includes EPA and DHA, which are essential for inflammation, heart health, and brain function. While plant sources like nuts and seeds contain ALA, a type of omega-3, it takes more effort for your body to convert ALA into EPA and DHA.

SOURCE OF OMEGA-3 FATTY ACIDS	APPROXIMATE CONTENT PER SERVING
Mackerel (3.5 oz.)	4,580 mg of EPA and DHA (combined)
Salmon (3.5 oz.)	2,150 mg of EPA and DHA (combined)
Anchovies (3.5 oz.)	2,053 mg of EPA and DHA (combined)
Sardines (3.5 oz.)	982 mg of EPA and DHA (combined)
Oysters (3.5 oz.)	391 mg of EPA and DHA (combined)
Chia seeds (1 oz.)	5,050 mg of ALA
Walnuts (1 oz.)	2,570 mg of ALA
Whole flaxseeds (0.35 oz., 1 tbsp)	2,350 mg of ALA

The Dietary Guidelines for Americans recommend eating at least 8 ounces of seafood per week (about two servings), prioritizing fatty fish like salmon, mackerel, sardines, and tuna to provide an average daily consumption of 250 milligrams of EPA and DHA.[41]

B VITAMINS

B vitamins are crucial for a lot of important functions in your body, like producing energy, supporting brain health, and keeping your nervous system healthy. They help convert food into energy, support the production of neurotransmitters that affect your mood, and play a role in maintaining healthy nerve function and the formation of red blood cells.

B vitamins can help decrease fatigue, particularly during times of increased energy demands or stress. They are also essential for the synthesis and metabolism of neurotransmitters.[42] Vitamins B6, folate (B9), and B12 are important for neurotransmitter synthesis, including serotonin, dopamine, and norepinephrine. Imbalances or deficiencies in these neurotransmitters have been linked to mood disorders such as depression and anxiety, which underscores the importance of adequate B vitamin intake for emotional well-being.[43]

B VITAMIN	FOOD SOURCE	
B1 (thiamine)	• fish • legumes • liver	• nuts and seeds • pork • yogurt
B2 (riboflavin)	• beef • chicken • dairy products • eggs • leafy green vegetables	• liver • meat • mushrooms • pork
B3 (niacin)	• bananas • beef • beef liver • fish	• legumes • pork • whole grains
B5 (pantothenic acid)	• avocados • beef • chicken • dairy milk • fish	• mushrooms • organ meats (liver, kidney) • whole grains
B6 (pyridoxine)	• bananas • beef liver • chicken • chickpeas	• potatoes • salmon • tuna
B7 (biotin)	• avocados • eggs • mushrooms • nuts and seeds	• organ meats (liver, kidney) • salmon • sweet potatoes

B9 (folate)	• asparagus • avocados • beetroot • broccoli • citrus fruits	• eggs • leafy green vegetables • legumes • liver • papaya
B12 (cobalamin)	• beef • chicken • clams • dairy products • eggs	• organ meat (liver, kidney) • salmon • sardines • tuna

A vitamin B complex supplement could be beneficial for those who have difficulty obtaining sufficient B vitamins from their diet alone, particularly vegans and vegetarians. This supplement can also be beneficial for those experiencing low energy and fatigue, which is common in those with low cortisol levels.

B vitamins are water soluble, meaning they do not accumulate in the body, and so the risk of toxicity is minimal. However, excessive intake of vitamin B6 may lead to neurological issues and should be avoided.

When selecting a B complex, look for supplements that contain highly absorbable forms of B vitamins, including methylcobalamin and 5-MTHF. These forms ensure optimal absorption and use, especially for people with genetic variations like an MTHFR gene variant. Always consult with a healthcare professional before starting any new supplement.

What food sources of vitamin C, magnesium, omega-3 fatty acids, and B vitamins could you add to your diet in light of what you've learned? Take a look at the lists again and try to include a few of these foods in your meals each day and fatty fish at least once a week.

• • •

Congratulations, you've completed Step One: Eat a Nutrient-Dense Diet! You now have a clear understanding of how to build nutrient-dense meals, including protein, fiber-rich carbs, and healthy fats. You also know which foods to avoid or limit in order to reduce inflammation, and you've got simple swaps in mind to make the transition smoother. Plus, you're well aware of the key nutrients and food sources that will support your stress response and help build resilience. You've really set yourself up for success! I know it feels like a lot to take in, so before progressing to Step Two, ensure you've given yourself lots of time to integrate everything you've learned in this chapter. To make it easier to put into practice, check out the recipe section in Part III (see page 261)—it's full of delicious ideas that bring these principles to life. And if you're curious about further nutritional support, turn to Appendix C (page 323), where I share information on adaptogenic herbs, known as "adaptogens," and other nutritional compounds that can support your resilience to stress.

Key Habits to Incorporate in Step One

Below, I've included a checklist to give you an idea of how you can make small weekly changes that all add up. Of course, feel free to adapt the suggestions to fit your lifestyle and progress at a pace that works best for you.

Week 1

This week is about building mindfulness when you eat and ensuring your meals include the right balance of macronutrients.

☐ Practice mindful eating at lunch.

☐ Ensure each of your main meals include at least 25 grams of protein.

☐ Include fiber-rich complex carbohydrates in each meal.

☐ Include high-quality fats in each meal.

Week 2

This week, you can add two new layers:

1. Swap inflammatory foods for better alternatives.
2. Incorporate foods rich in key nutrients that support the HPA axis.

☐ Continue with the habits from Week 1, but expand mindful eating to dinner as well.

☐ Identify at least one inflammatory food you regularly eat and swap it for a better alternative (for example, replace a store-bought cookie with a square of dark chocolate).

☐ If applicable to you and with the supervision of your doctor or dietitian, eliminate foods you are sensitive to.

☐ Add a source of polyphenols (for example, berries or green tea), prebiotics (for example, artichokes or oats), or probiotics (for example, yogurt, kefir, sauerkraut).

☐ Add nutrients that support your stress response, such as magnesium-rich foods like pumpkin seeds, spinach, or almonds; a source of vitamin C (for example, add camu camu powder to yogurt or a smoothie); and a source of omega-3 fatty acids (for example, fatty fish like salmon or sardines).

At the end of the 2 weeks, reflect on how these swaps and additions are making you feel. Maintain all your new habits and continue to build on them, for example, by swapping another inflammatory food (perhaps replacing white bread with whole-wheat or sourdough) and expanding mindful eating to breakfast so you are practicing it at all three meals. Once you feel confident in your understanding and you notice that these habits are becoming second nature, go back to pages 47–50 and do the questionnaires again—have you noticed a difference in any of the symptoms you identified before you started the plan?

You can now confidently move on to the next step: Balance Your Blood Sugar.

Step Two

Balance Your Blood Sugar

When diet is wrong, medicine is of no use. When diet is correct, medicine is of no need.

—AYURVEDIC PROVERB

Welcome to Step Two of the plan, where you will learn everything you need to know about achieving balanced blood sugar. We've already seen in Part I how constant wild fluctuations in blood sugar can have many long-term consequences, including not only weight gain and fatigue but also inflammation, oxidative stress, cortisol imbalances, dysregulation of the HPA axis, and more chances of developing chronic diseases like metabolic diseases, heart conditions, and even cancer. I often tell my clients to prioritize balancing their blood sugar levels as if their very life depended on it, because it truly does!

But what I find especially interesting is that symptoms of poor blood sugar regulation often mimic mental health symptoms such as anxiety, along with mood disturbances like irritability or mood swings. This connection is important for people with recurrent mental health symptoms, as maintaining stable blood sugar levels could significantly improve the way they feel.

I wasn't aware of my own blood sugar issues and how they were triggering my anxiety for years. Frankly, I thought only people diagnosed with insulin resistance or diabetes had problems regulating their blood sugar. This misconception couldn't be further from reality. One study found that just 1 in 8 adults in the United States has optimal metabolic health, including healthy glucose levels.[1] While this study focused on the United States, similar trends are emerging globally with rates of insulin resistance, metabolic syndrome, and type 2 diabetes on the rise.[2] This suggests that a significant portion of the global population is struggling with managing blood sugar without even realizing it.

This was me! Most of the symptoms I struggled with daily, such as anxiety, poor sleep, cravings, food obsession, and weakness if I waited too long between meals, were clear messages from my body. I was riding a blood sugar "roller coaster" of spikes and crashes. Let's quickly talk about what blood sugar spikes are to see if the symptoms resonate with you, too.

Understanding Blood Sugar Spikes

Blood sugar spikes happen when there is a rapid increase in blood glucose (sugar) levels. Typically, these spikes result from either consuming too many carbohydrates in general or eating certain foods that rapidly raise blood sugar, such as refined carbohydrates like white bread and rice, as well as simple sugars (found in table sugar, high-fructose corn syrup, honey, maple syrup, fruit juices, candy and other sweets, sugary drinks like soda or sweet tea, sweetened breakfast cereals, or ice cream). In other words, both the quantity and the type of carbohydrates are important factors in blood sugar spikes.

To provide context, according to the American Diabetes Association, normal fasting blood sugar levels (before you eat) should be under 100 mg/dL (5.6 mmol/L).[3] After you eat, blood sugar levels are going to naturally increase, and this is normal, but both the International Diabetes Federation and the American Diabetes Association recommend keeping post-meal glucose levels below 140 mg/dL (7.8 mmol/L) when measured 1 to 2 hours after the start of a meal.[4]

When blood sugar rises above this threshold after eating, it is often considered a blood sugar spike. Repeated spikes contribute to greater glucose *variability*, which research suggests may increase the risk of complications related to diabetes and overall metabolic health.[5]

As we've seen, a spike in glucose triggers a surge in insulin production. In some cases, this can cause too much glucose to be cleared from the bloodstream, leading to a "crash" or even hypoglycemia (see page 38). And since low blood sugar is a powerful trigger for the stress response, this up-and-down pattern can feel especially draining.

Over time, frequent insulin surges can cause the body's cells to become less responsive—a process called insulin resistance. This means glucose remains in the bloodstream for longer, raising blood sugar levels and increasing the risk of developing type 2 diabetes and other metabolic issues.

Problems maintaining optimal blood sugar levels have been linked to fatigue, anxiety, irritability, cravings, migraines, sleep disturbances, inflammation, increased risk of chronic diseases such as cardiovascular disease, diabetes and obesity, hormonal imbalances and fertility issues (such as polycystic ovary syndrome—PCOS), brain fog, mood swings, and even accelerated ageing.[6]

Once you master the art of stabilizing your blood sugar and decreasing blood sugar variability, you will experience transformative benefits, often in a short period of time, including more energy, less anxiety, a more stable mood, better concentration, fewer cravings, better weight management, and more regular menstrual cycles. And, even more importantly, learning to manage your blood sugar will help you avoid unnecessarily triggering the stress response and the release of cortisol. Over time, this creates a ripple effect: It reduces strain on your system, helps reduce inflammation, and supports your cells in producing energy more efficiently—building the foundation for long-term stress resilience.

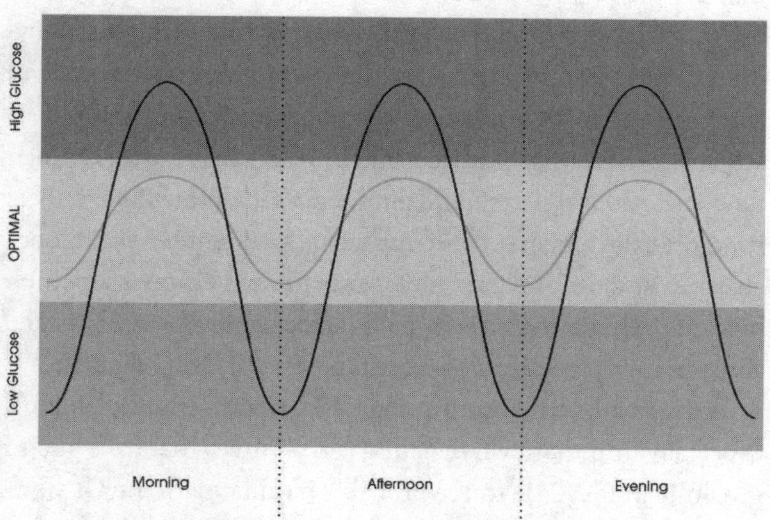

Blood glucose levels throughout the day: Stable (optimal, gray line) versus the variable (highs and lows, black line).

Now that you've seen how important it is to reduce blood sugar variability to build your stress resilience, let's look at how you actually do that, revisiting those macronutrients we met in Step One!

Embrace the Trio: Protein, Carbohydrates, and Fat

The first strategy for improving blood sugar balance and avoiding spikes and crashes is to *consistently* pair carbohydrates with protein and fat. We explored this when we looked at building a nutrient-dense diet in Step One, but this principle is also key here, and the great news is that the habits you've already established are helping you manage your blood sugar more effectively.

When we consume carbohydrates alone, especially those that are rapidly absorbed, this can cause a sudden spike in blood glucose levels. However, when we combine carbohydrates with protein and fat, the digestion process slows down, leading to a more gradual release of glucose into the bloodstream. The rate of gastric emptying, or the speed at which food leaves the stomach and enters the small intestine, affects how quickly glucose from digested food enters the bloodstream. Protein and fat slow down gastric emptying, which helps to reduce the rise in blood glucose levels after meals. This, in turn, can also help moderate the insulin response.[7]

Pairing carbs with protein and fat is always beneficial, but it's especially important when eating carb sources that have a high glycemic index (GI). You're probably familiar with the GI since some diets are built around the concept of avoiding or limiting foods high in the GI to improve blood sugar balance. The GI of food measures how quickly carbohydrates in that food raise blood glucose levels compared to pure glucose. Foods with a high GI value lead to a rapid surge in blood sugar levels and insulin and may be followed by a sharp decline in blood sugar. On the other hand, foods with a low GI value are digested and absorbed more gradually, resulting in a slower rise in blood sugar levels and insulin, which leads to a more stable decline of blood sugar over time. Examples of high-GI foods are white rice, rice crackers, white bread, pastries, and sweetened breakfast cereals. Examples of foods with lower GI are rolled oats, pears, apples or berries, beans, and non-starchy vegetables.

Interestingly, while protein and fat don't have a GI value, they influence the overall glycemic impact of the meal by delaying gastric emptying.[8] Beyond their impact on blood sugar, protein and fat also keep you feeling full and satisfied for longer, which will help you achieve better weight control.

Let me show you how effective pairing carbohydrates with protein and fat is with a real-life example. Mary, a 53-year-old woman, was struggling with fatigue, intense cravings for sweets, and weight gain. We made some changes to Mary's meals to make sure they included a combination of carbohydrates, protein, and healthy fats. For example, instead of her usual bowl of cornflakes with sliced banana and oat milk for breakfast, we introduced options including:

- cottage cheese with mixed berries, plus nuts or seeds
- oatmeal made with rolled oats, milk, and protein powder, topped with sliced almonds
- avocado toast on whole-grain bread, paired with scrambled eggs and a chicken sausage

For lunch, we moved away from her usual sandwich with white bread or veggie wrap with little protein, and chose meals like:

- grilled chicken salad with mixed greens, quinoa, and extra-virgin olive oil dressing
- savory cottage cheese bowl with chopped cucumbers, tomatoes, and peppers, topped with herbs and pistachios
- tuna salad with leafy greens, cucumber, avocado, and a drizzle of extra-virgin olive oil

For dinner, instead of her typical takeout, we kept it simple with options like:

- one-pan roasted salmon and roasted veggies
- a homemade beef chili with black beans and a side of steamed broccoli
- shrimp stir-fry with mixed vegetables and buckwheat noodles

The impact of these changes became evident through Mary's continuous glucose monitor readings. Previously, she had experienced spikes in her blood sugar levels, often peaking at around 150 mg/dL (8.3 mmol/L), or even higher after some meals—followed by crashes that left her feeling tired and triggering cravings. However, by making sure that all her meals consisted of a balanced combination of carbohydrates with protein and fat, her blood sugar levels stabilized overnight, with fewer spikes and less dramatic drops.

Her glucose after her meals is now consistently down to under 125 mg/dL (7 mmol/L) which shows how effective it is to balance your meals with a good ratio of protein, carbs, and fat. More importantly, though, her symptoms improved in a matter of days. She started feeling a lot more energetic, with fewer cravings for sweets, and started losing some of that extra weight she was struggling with.

Given what you've just learned, are there some changes you can make to your daily meals to ensure you are pairing carbohydrates with protein and fat? This step may already be well covered given the habits you've introduced from Step One, but take a moment to see if there's anything you can tweak to ensure you're consistently combining all three macronutrients—carbs, protein, and fat—at each meal. Revisit the meal planner you completed on page 93, and remember, there are recipes for breakfast, lunch, and dinner in Part III (page 261), which all have a good balance of the three macronutrients.

Adding protein and fat to your carbohydrates is going to help you improve blood sugar regulation, but there's another key player that shouldn't be overlooked: fiber!

Make Sure You Get Enough Fiber

Fiber is a type of carbohydrate found in plant-based foods. Unlike other carbohydrates, fiber can't be broken down, so it passes through the digestive system relatively intact, meaning that it isn't broken down into glucose. Studies show that fiber has many health benefits and can decrease your risk of cardiovascular disease, diabetes, and cancer.[9] The recommended daily fiber intake for adults up to age fifty is 25 grams for women and 38 grams for men, according to the USDA.[10] For adults over fifty, the recommended amounts are 21 grams for women and 30 grams for men. However, most people fall short of these guidelines, with average intakes around 16 grams of fiber per day.[11]

Fiber can be soluble and insoluble, and while both types of fiber have beneficial effects, soluble fiber is particularly helpful because it forms a gel-like substance when combined with water that slows down the absorption of glucose into the bloodstream.

Foods high in soluble fiber include oats, barley, legumes (such as black beans, kidney beans, navy beans, lentils, and chickpeas), fruits (like avocados, figs, kiwi, bananas, berries, apples, oranges, and pears), vegetables (such as artichokes, Brussel sprouts, carrots, sweet potatoes, broccoli, and asparagus), and psyllium husk.

Foods high in insoluble fiber include whole grains (like whole-wheat bread, quinoa, and brown rice), legumes (as above), nuts and seeds (such as almonds, walnuts, and sunflower seeds), vegetables (such as leafy greens, cauliflower, and green beans), and fruits with edible skins (like apples, pears, and plums).

When it comes to benefits regarding blood sugar regulation, one review of multiple studies showed that higher fiber intake is linked to better glycemic control, with reductions in HbA1c (the average level of blood sugar over the past 2 to 3 months), fasting glucose, insulin levels, and insulin resistance, as well as reductions in inflammation and improvements in cholesterol and triglyceride levels.[12]

Let's compare the impact on glucose of eating an orange versus drinking orange juice. When you eat a whole orange, you're consuming not just the fruit's natural sugars but also its fiber content. The fiber in the orange slows down digestion, which leads to a more gradual release of glucose into the bloodstream, leading to a slower rise in blood sugar. In contrast, orange juice is a concentrated source of the fruit's sugars without the accompanying fiber. Without fiber to slow down digestion, the sugars in the juice are rapidly absorbed, leading to a quick spike in blood sugar levels.

But that's not all! Fiber can also improve insulin sensitivity, which is key when it comes to efficient blood sugar management.[13] Remember that insulin is the hormone your pancreas secretes to facilitate the absorption of glucose by the cells. However, when insulin is constantly high, cells start to become less and less responsive to it (known as insulin resistance), which can hinder the absorption by the cells and leave too much glucose in the blood. By improving insulin sensitivity, fiber helps cells to take glucose more effectively, decreasing the risk of developing insulin resistance and type 2 diabetes.[14]

And let's not forget the beneficial effects that fiber has on the ecosystem in the gut: the microbiome we met in Step One (see page 79). Some types of fiber act as prebiotics that "feed" beneficial bacteria in the gut, helping it grow. These beneficial bacteria ferment prebiotics into SCFAs. These SCFAs are called "postbiotics" and have been shown to decrease inflammation and improve metabolic health.[15]

SOURCE OF FIBER	APPROXIMATE FIBER CONTENT PER SERVING
Black beans (½ cup, cooked)	9 g
Split peas (½ cup, cooked)	8 g
Lentils (½ cup, cooked)	8 g
Chickpeas (½ cup, cooked)	8 g
Artichoke (1 medium)	7 g
Raspberries (½ cup)	4 g
Avocado (½ medium)	6.5 g
Pear (1 medium with skin)	5.5 g
Psyllium husk (1 tbsp)	5 g
Apple (1 medium with skin)	4.5 g
Chia seeds (1 tbsp)	4 g
Brussels sprouts (½ cup, cooked)	3.8 g
Almonds (1 oz.)	3.8 g
Sweet potato (1 medium cooked with skin)	3.3 g
Banana (1 medium)	3 g
Sunflower seeds (1 oz.)	3 g
Oats (½ cup, cooked)	3 g
Quinoa (½ cup, cooked)	2.8 g
Spinach (½ cup, cooked)	2.7 g
Broccoli (½ cup, cooked)	2.6 g
Carrot (1 large, raw)	2.5 g
Flaxseeds, ground (1 tbsp)	2 g
Strawberries (½ cup)	1.5 g

Incorporating fiber-rich foods into your daily diet is a powerful strategy for reducing the physical stress that blood sugar spikes place on the body, decreasing inflammation, and preventing unnecessary activation of the stress response and excess cortisol release. The good news is that if you've been following the principles from Step One—choosing whole, minimally processed foods, such as fruits, vegetables, legumes, whole grains, nuts, and seeds—you've likely already increased your fiber intake!

Take a look at the list above: Are you already including some of these fiber-rich foods daily? If not, start by gradually adding more. Just be mindful to increase your intake slowly, as a sudden jump from low to high fiber can cause digestive discomfort. And don't forget to drink plenty of water throughout the day to help keep things moving smoothly!

Below are a few examples of how to introduce more fiber-rich foods to your diet this week:

BREAKFAST	• Try rolled oats for breakfast. Cook them in water or milk and mix in protein powder for a balanced meal. You can also make overnight oats with Greek yogurt or stir cooked oats into cottage cheese (see recipe on page 264). • Add psyllium husk to a big glass of water or your smoothie. • Top your yogurt with raspberries and a few almonds. • Swap white bread for whole grain.
LUNCH AND DINNER	• Add any type of bean (lentils, chickpeas, black beans) to salads or soups. • Include a variety of vegetables in every meal—aim for half your plate to be non-starchy veggies. • Swap white rice for quinoa, farro or whole-grain options. • Choose whole-grain wraps, pasta, or crackers instead of refined versions. • If organic, leave the skin on fruits and vegetables where possible (for example, apples, cucumbers, potatoes).
SNACKS	• Enjoy nuts, seeds, or hummus with veggie sticks. • Eat whole fruits instead of drinking fruit juices.

Now that you understand why creating balanced meals with fiber-rich carbs, protein, and fat can support your blood sugar balance, let's take it up a notch.

Don't Skip Breakfast

I am a big advocate for eating breakfast, but not just any breakfast—a balanced breakfast with plenty of protein! Opting for a quick fix like a cup of coffee and a banana (which doesn't seem that bad) because you're not that hungry can set the stage for a blood sugar roller-coaster ride. On the other hand, starting your day with a high-protein breakfast not only prevents immediate spikes but has been shown to improve satiety and appetite control for the rest of the day.[16]

Interestingly, eating breakfast has also been shown to reinforce the circadian rhythm, influencing genes that support metabolic processes like insulin sensitivity, helping to maintain more stable blood sugar levels throughout the day. Skipping breakfast, on the other hand, might disrupt these genes and lead to higher blood sugar levels after meals.[17]

You might be thinking, "But isn't fasting good for you?" The short answer is yes, for some people. While fasting has been extensively researched and shown to offer plenty of benefits, it might not be suitable for everyone.[18] Much of the research doesn't account for the differences in metabolism between men and women, as well as the hormonal fluctuations that occur throughout the menstrual cycle in women. In my experience, women who already have hormonal imbalances or are dealing with high levels of stress may not experience the same benefits from fasting.

In fact, for many, and for women in particular, skipping breakfast can add another layer of stress to their already overloaded systems. Take my client Priya. Seeing her husband reap the benefits of fasting, she decided to follow suit. However, despite following the exact same fasting routine as her husband, eating only in an 8-hour window each day, Priya barely lost any weight. Even worse, she noticed a decline in her mood and energy levels. Every day, as the clock ticked toward 10 and 11 a.m., Priya started feeling increasingly cranky and anxious, which disrupted her focus and productivity at work. By the time lunch came around, she was ravenous and often overate, which left her bloated and tired.

Priya's husband was thriving on his fasting routine. He lost a considerable amount of weight fairly quickly, and he felt energetic and more focused. This made Priya even more frustrated and confused. Why wasn't she experiencing similar benefits?

Fasting, or long periods without eating, causes a drop in blood sugar and triggers the release of glucocorticoids such as cortisol. While these help to raise blood sugar levels to maintain energy balance, chronic elevation of cortisol levels, as we know, can be problematic. This is why having breakfast is crucial—it's another of those "low-hanging fruits" that will give your body's stress response a much-needed break. By starting the day with a balanced meal, you can stabilize your blood sugar levels, support hormonal balance, and reduce the burden on your body's stress response system.

When Priya switched gears and prioritized having a nutrient-dense breakfast comprising plenty of protein, plus fiber-rich carbs and fats—her favorites were the Pre- and Probiotic Smoothie (page 266) and the Egg and Black Bean Breakfast Taco (page 267)—rather than fasting, she quickly noticed improvements in her health and well-being. Not only did she achieve better energy, reduced cravings, and an improved mood, she also effortlessly shed a few pounds!

If you find you're not hungry in the morning, try eating a smaller breakfast or consider adjusting the size of your dinner the night before so you are hungrier when you wake up. In fact, making your breakfast and lunch bigger meals compared to dinner has been shown to lead to better glucose control, reduced hunger, and improved satiety.[19] Try it this week and see if it makes a difference in how you feel.

Maintain Consistent Mealtimes

Once you're in the habit of eating a high-protein breakfast every day, consistency in meal timing is the next factor in maintaining stable blood sugar levels throughout the day. Striking the right balance between meal frequency and spacing is crucial. As we've just seen, too many hours between meals can lead to blood sugar dips. On the other hand, constant grazing or snacking disrupts your body's natural rhythm and insulin response. The key is to opt for consistent meals at regular intervals.

Below is a sample meal schedule to help you maintain consistency throughout the day:

- breakfast: 7:30 a.m.
- lunch: 12:00 p.m.
- afternoon snack (optional): 3:00 p.m.
- dinner: 6:30 p.m.

Adjust these times based on your individual schedule and preferences, but strive to maintain a consistent pattern of eating to support stable blood sugar levels and overall metabolic health.

Remember: There's no need to overhaul your meal schedule all at once. Start by aiming to have breakfast at the same time each day, then gradually do the same for lunch and dinner. Over time, your body will adjust and naturally start to expect food at the same times.

By sticking to a consistent meal schedule, you will also support your circadian rhythm. I will explain how this works in more detail in Step Three (page 144), but for now, know that eating at regular times supports optimal metabolic function and helps regulate your blood sugar levels more effectively.

Once you've mastered these new habits, you can move on to the next habit that will help you achieve better blood sugar control, enhance satiety, and promote overall metabolic health.

Move Your Body

It's not just what you eat that affects your blood sugar levels; how much or how little you move your body can also have an impact. When we engage in physical activity, the muscles contract and this activates glucose transporters that allow the cells to take in glucose from the bloodstream *without* needing insulin. Imagine every muscle contraction as a fleet of trucks picking up glucose and delivering it to the power plants (mitochondria) for energy production.

The insulin-like effect of muscle contraction can help to stabilize blood sugar levels while minimizing insulin release, which is beneficial because it helps to maintain optimal insulin levels.[20] Remember that we don't want to have constant high levels of insulin, as high insulin levels (hyperinsulinemia) can eventually lead to insulin resistance.

When I talk about muscle contraction, I'm not referring only to traditional exercise such as running or swimming. *Any type of movement* can contribute to better blood sugar management. In fact, a systematic review showed that even just standing up frequently for short periods significantly lowered glucose levels after meals compared to sitting. Light-intensity walking was even more effective in reducing glucose spikes and maintaining stable insulin levels.[21] A study in people with type 2 diabetes found that taking a light 10-minute walk after each meal was more effective for blood sugar management than a single 30-minute walk at any other time of day.[22]

Brianna, one of my clients, had been dealing with fatigue, brain fog, and concentration issues at work. After making changes to her meals by adding more protein and fiber, she started to feel more focused and energized. However, the fatigue after lunch still lingered. So she decided to incorporate a simple 15-minute walk after her midday meal. After just a few days, Brianna noticed significant improvements. Not only did her post-lunch fatigue improve, but she also felt more alert and focused throughout the afternoon. She even mentioned feeling calmer, likely because she was spending 15 minutes walking through the park in a natural setting. I'll explain in Step Five (page 199) how spending a few minutes in nature, even in green urban spaces, can have a powerful impact on our mental health. If you feel that some of the symptoms of poor blood sugar regulation are lingering, such as fatigue, cravings, weight gain, brain fog, irritability, or anxiety, try introducing some movement into your day, like Brianna, to support the other habits you have introduced.

More intense exercise like aerobic activities and resistance training can bring significant benefits for long-term blood sugar management and metabolic health as well as increase stress resilience. While more moderate and intense exercise triggers cortisol production, it has been shown to dampen the cortisol response to subsequent perceived stressors. This helps improve the body's ability to manage stress more effectively over time.[23] In Step Four, we'll dive into the specifics of exercise and its impact on stress, exploring various workout strategies and how to seamlessly weave them into your daily routine.

I know that, for some of you with busy lives, it's hard to see how you can incorporate even simple movement into your day. So, here's a practical example of how you can easily implement just 10 minutes of movement into your everyday routine: After a meal, ideally about 30 minutes after, take a 10-minute walk around the block. If walking isn't possible, consider using the stairs, doing squats, or simply standing up every half hour instead of sitting down. Remember, any movement is better than no movement. The goal is to stimulate muscle contractions that will increase glucose uptake, preventing spikes in blood sugar after meals.

Harness Nutrients and Foods That Support Blood Sugar Balance

You've worked hard in this step to balance your blood sugar and hopefully you're starting to see the benefits of creating balanced meals with fiber-rich carbs, protein, and fat, as well as the importance of not skipping meals, especially breakfast, and the benefits of moving after your meals. Now, let's dive into a few nutrients—magnesium, chromium, vitamin D, B vitamins, alpha-lipoic acid, and inositol—that have been shown to support blood sugar regulation, as well as cinnamon and other polyphenol-rich foods, such as green tea, that contain bioactive compounds that can stabilize blood sugar levels and improve insulin sensitivity.

The research in this area is promising and, when combined with the other strategies discussed in this step, might further improve your metabolic health and overall well-being.

MAGNESIUM

Magnesium plays a key role in energy metabolism and glucose transport across cell membranes, and not having enough of it can disrupt the insulin receptor's activity inside cells, which can lead to reduced insulin sensitivity. Low magnesium levels have been associated with insulin resistance, impaired glucose tolerance, and increased risk of type 2 diabetes.[24] By ensuring an adequate intake of magnesium-rich foods (see page 112) and potentially including a magnesium supplement if needed (see pages 112–13), you can support optimal glucose metabolism and insulin sensitivity.

CHROMIUM

Chromium might improve the action of insulin and facilitates the absorption of glucose into cells. Chromium picolinate, specifically, has been shown to reduce insulin resistance and the risk of cardiovascular disease and type 2 diabetes.[25] Including chromium-rich foods like whole grains, broccoli, green beans, brewer's yeast, beef, turkey, fish, and apples in your diet can support healthy blood sugar levels.

VITAMIN D

Vitamin D plays a role in improving insulin sensitivity. It improves the production and secretion of insulin while also promoting glucose uptake by cells. Vitamin D deficiency has been associated with insulin resistance and impaired glucose metabolism, increasing the risk of type 2 diabetes.[26] Eating vitamin D–rich foods like fatty fish, mushrooms, and eggs, and getting adequate sunlight exposure can help maintain optimal vitamin D levels and support blood sugar regulation.

B VITAMINS

B vitamins are closely related to blood sugar regulation, as they help support processes involved in energy metabolism. Some B vitamins, such as B6, B9, and B12, influence glucose metabolism and the action of insulin. Eating foods rich in B vitamins (see pages 115–16) can help maintain optimal energy metabolism and blood sugar balance.

ALPHA-LIPOIC ACID

Alpha-lipoic acid is an antioxidant that can help lower blood sugar levels and improve insulin sensitivity. Research suggests that alpha-lipoic acid supplementation may improve glucose tolerance and insulin sensitivity in people with insulin resistance or type 2 diabetes.[27] Organ meats, red meat, broccoli, tomatoes, spinach, and Brussels sprouts are good sources.

INOSITOL

Inositol plays a role in cellular signaling and insulin sensitivity, both of which are important for good blood sugar regulation. The best food sources are fruits like cantaloupe, citrus fruits (especially oranges), beans, whole grains, nuts, seeds, and organ meats. Research suggests that inositol supplementation can improve glycemic control in conditions such as insulin resistance and PCOS, mitigating the risk of hyperglycemia and related metabolic disorders.[28] There are many forms of inositol, but the two that have the biggest impact on PCOS are myo-inositol and D-chiro-inositol.

CINNAMON

Cinnamon is not only delicious, but it also offers benefits for blood sugar regulation. It contains compounds that might improve insulin sensitivity and help lower blood sugar levels.

One study of 80 people with PCOS found that taking 1.5 grams of cinnamon powder daily for 12 weeks caused a significant reduction in fasting insulin levels and improved insulin sensitivity compared with a placebo.[29] Another study found that taking 250 milligrams of cinnamon twice daily for 2 months improved insulin sensitivity in 137 people with high blood sugar levels.[30]

If you are going to regularly eat cinnamon, try to get Ceylon cinnamon rather than cassia, because Ceylon cinnamon has lower levels of coumarin, a compound that may be harmful in large doses, and so it is a safer and healthier option for regular consumption.

You can add cinnamon to oatmeal, yogurt, or smoothies for a tasty and blood sugar–friendly boost. It's also available in herbal teas, or you can create your own by simply simmering 3 cinnamon sticks in 2 cups of water for about 5–10 minutes.

POLYPHENOL-RICH FOODS

We met polyphenols in Step One for their ability to improve gut bacteria and support gut health (see page 105). Hopefully, you've already incorporated many of these sources into your diet. Now, we're going to focus on how they can also support blood sugar regulation.

Remember that polyphenols are naturally occurring compounds found in plants. Some of the richest sources include berries such as blueberries, blackberries, raspberries, and strawberries, along with apples, grapes, pomegranates, and cherries. Vegetables like red onions, spinach, and artichokes are also excellent sources. Drinks such as coffee, green tea, and black tea are particularly high in polyphenols, as are cocoa and dark chocolate. Additional sources include spices (see Cinnamon on page 140), olives, extra-virgin olive oil, soy, nuts, and seeds.

Studies suggest that polyphenols might help lower blood sugar through several potential mechanisms, such as inhibiting enzymes that break down carbohydrates,[31] reducing blood sugar spikes. They can also increase insulin sensitivity and improve glucose uptake in cells. Additionally, polyphenols have antioxidant properties that help prevent oxidative stress, which supports better blood sugar control.[32]

Among polyphenols, those found in berries, cherries, purple vegetables, green tea, coffee, extra-virgin olive oil, and cinnamon (see above) can be particularly effective in improving blood sugar control.

Think about which of these foods rich in nutrients you could introduce to support blood sugar management.

• • •

Congratulations on completing Step Two: Balance Your Blood Sugar! As I mentioned in "How the Cortisol Reset Plan Will Help You Thrive," I suggest taking at least 2 weeks to integrate the new habits you've learned into your daily routine before moving on to the next step.

Key Habits to Incorporate in Step Two

Below is a checklist with suggestions for how you can make small changes over the next 2 weeks. Again, feel free to adapt this to reflect the pace that works best for you.

Week 3

Continue building on the habits you established in Step One, and start progressively introducing the new habits you've learned in this step over the next 2 weeks.

- ☐ Ensure you are always pairing protein and fat with your carbs, even for snacks. Refer to the lists of protein sources (pages 73–74), carbohydrates sources (pages 82–84), and fat sources (pages 89–91), or to Part III for meal ideas (page 261).
- ☐ Introduce more fiber to your breakfast (page 131). For example, try rolled oats for breakfast (see the Blueberry and Cottage Cheese Oatmeal recipe on page 264) or add some nuts or seeds to your yogurt bowl. Try adding beans to your salad or soup for lunch or dinner.
- ☐ Make sure you eat a balanced breakfast with plenty of protein every day.
- ☐ Introduce foods rich in nutrients that support blood sugar management (see page 137). For example, you could have spinach or broccoli (sources of chromium) with fatty fish and mushrooms (rich in B vitamins and vitamin D).

Week 4

This week, you'll continue with the habits from Weeks 1–3, but also focus on maintaining a consistent meal schedule, introducing some movement into your days, and incorporating nutrients and foods that support blood sugar balance.

- ☐ Create a meal schedule and, from now on, try to eat all your meals at more or less the same time.
- ☐ Add a short walk or 10-minute movement session (go up and down the stairs, do some squats, or engage in light housework) after lunch.
- ☐ Eat polyphenol-rich foods every day. For example, eat a handful of blueberries or have a cup of green tea.
- ☐ Introduce foods rich in nutrients that support blood sugar management, such as spinach and kale (rich in magnesium); broccoli and green beans (sources of chromium); fatty fish and mushrooms (high in vitamin D); meat, fish, dairy, and eggs (high in B vitamins); as well as foods containing alpha-lipoic acid, such as spinach and broccoli, and inositol, found in cantaloupe melon, buckwheat, and citrus fruits.

Once you notice that these habits are becoming second nature, take them one step further—perhaps by adding a short walk after lunch *and* dinner or adding cinnamon to your yogurt or oats in the morning. Now, go back to pages 47–50 and do the questionnaires again: Is there any change in your symptoms?

Proceed to Step Three when you feel confident that these habits are firmly established. It's time to discover one of the best ways to address HPA axis dysfunction and cortisol imbalances: with circadian rhythm regulation.

Step Three

Regulate Your Circadian Rhythm

Keep your face always toward the sunshine—and shadows will fall behind you.

—COMMONLY ATTRIBUTED TO WALT WHITMAN

In the first two steps, we focused a lot on the foods you eat and how, with some small and consistent changes, you can reduce common stressors, balance cortisol levels, and build your energy reserves—ultimately boosting your stress resilience. Now, we're going to shift our attention to regulating your body's internal clock.

If you've ever travelled across multiple time zones, you're likely familiar with the dreaded "jet lag": feeling tired during the day, lying awake at night, battling mental fog and mood swings, dealing with an erratic appetite and a disrupted bathroom schedule, and just a general sensation of feeling "off." At the core of these symptoms is a misalignment in your circadian rhythm.

Think of your circadian rhythm as your body's internal clock that not only regulates your sleep–wake cycle but also most physiological processes, including metabolism, digestion, immune function, hormone balance, cognitive function, and more. When this rhythm is disrupted, whether by working night shifts, caring for a newborn, frequent travel, erratic sleep habits, or other factors, it can leave you feeling exhausted, moody, and unable to function at your best. Over time, these disruptions can lead to more serious issues.

Studies indicate that people who do shift work (one of the most common disruptors of the circadian rhythm) are more likely to develop health issues such as gut problems, obesity, diabetes, and cardiovascular diseases compared to those with regular schedules.[1]

While jet lag and shift work are obvious examples of circadian disruptors, there are more subtle ways to throw off our circadian rhythm. These are often linked to our tendency to pack more and more into our day, like work, bingeing on Netflix, phone scrolling, and other activities, all at the expense of our sleep.

We touched on circadian disruption and how important the circadian system is in maintaining homeostasis and optimal health in Part I. Before we look at the habits you can introduce to regulate your circadian rhythm, I want to just dive a little bit deeper into how the circadian rhythm works so you understand why it's so important for your health.

Understanding Your Internal Clock

Everything that your body does needs to be done at a specific time to make sure the whole system works smoothly. Almost every cell in your body contains a circadian clock—known as "peripheral clocks"—that control the expression of certain genes, turning them on and off in a specific sequence, influencing things like hormone release, metabolism, your immune system, and more.[2] This careful timing ensures that sleep, digestion, growth, and tissue repair happen at the best times for efficiency.

The peripheral clocks need to be synchronized with the external environment through external cues called *zeitgebers*, which is a German word meaning "time givers" or "timekeepers." Light is the most powerful zeitgeber, but two other important cues are meal timing and physical activity. Much like a clock that isn't regularly reset, our peripheral clocks can begin to drift if they are not consistently *aligned* with the external environment. This process, known as "entrainment," ensures that our internal rhythms align with the 24-hour day.

The key player in entrainment is the suprachiasmatic nucleus (SCN), often referred to as the "master clock." This small part of the brain receives input from the eyes through cells that are highly sensitive to light (these are called "retinal ganglion cells"). These cells detect changes in light intensity and wavelength (day–night cycle) and send this info to the SCN. The SCN then communicates with other parts of the brain and body using neural, hormonal (melatonin, cortisol), and molecular signals to synchronize the peripheral clocks with the 24-hour cycle.

For example, peripheral clocks in your digestive tract control when to release hormones like ghrelin (the hunger hormone) and leptin (the satiety hormone), when to produce digestive enzymes, absorb nutrients, and move food and waste through the digestive system. The clock in the pancreas times when to produce insulin or slow down production. Each peripheral clock operates independently, but they all need to be synchronized with the 24-hour cycle.

Without this adjustment, our internal clocks would drift out of sync with the natural day–night cycle, leading to circadian rhythm disruption, which can have significant effects on our overall health. Circadian disruption increases allostatic load, affecting cognitive function, mood, and physical health.[3] This is a major stressor for the body and a recognized leading cause of HPA axis dysfunction and cortisol dysregulation. In fact, the timing of cortisol release (the daily pattern we discussed in Part I, page 27) is influenced by the circadian system, particularly the SCN and its interaction with the HPA axis.

To optimize our health and build and maintain resilience to stress and disease, our job is to ensure that our internal clocks are synchronized with the environment and the 24-hour day–night cycle. In this step, I'll show how you can do that by reinforcing the three key timekeeping signals: light exposure, meal timing, and physical activity, as well as optimizing sleep quality, which is one of the most important ways your body stays in sync with its natural circadian rhythms.

I recognize that many of the strategies I will discuss in this chapter may not be fully feasible for those of you working shift jobs. However, I have shared some tips on pages 158–59 that can help minimize the disruptive effects of shift work on your circadian rhythm.

Master Light Exposure

For most plants and animals, including humans, light is the most important external clue that helps sync our circadian rhythm with the day–night cycle. Exposure to light (blue light, in particular) stimulates the retinal ganglion cells, which then send signals to the SCN. The timing and duration of light exposure can either support and reinforce the circadian rhythm or disrupt it, acting as a circadian disruptor.

Humans evolved without electricity, and their daily activities were entirely driven by sunlight. They would wake up at sunrise, exposed to bright, blue-rich light that sent a clear signal to the brain (through the eyes) that the day had begun. As the day progressed, exposure to daylight kept them alert and productive. When evening arrived and the sun set, the gradual decrease of light intensity and onset of darkness provided a clear signal to their brain that the day was ending, prompting the body to prepare for rest and sleep.

The way we live today is a lot different, creating challenges for our circadian rhythm, which remains the same as our ancestors. The use of artificial lighting, such as indoor lighting and electronic devices that emit blue light, can confuse our SCN by receiving light inputs at all times of the day. For example, exposure to artificial light in the evening, particularly from screens in smartphones, tablets, computers, and TVs, can suppress the production of melatonin, the hormone that regulates the sleep–wake cycle. This suppression can delay the onset of sleep and interfere with the quality and duration of sleep.[4] Similarly, irregular sleep schedules, shift work, and social jet lag (such as staying up later on weekends compared to weekdays) can disrupt our circadian rhythms by exposing us to light at inappropriate times and altering our sleep patterns.

Though it's not realistic to eliminate artificial light, understanding how light affects you can help you make meaningful changes. By adopting a few simple habits, you can adjust your light exposure to better align with your natural rhythms.

EXPOSE YOUR EYES TO SUNLIGHT IN THE MORNING

Morning sunlight is rich in blue light, which stimulates specialized photoreceptors in the retina that are particularly sensitive to the short-wavelength light typical of the morning. When activated, these photoreceptors send strong signals to the SCN, which then synchronizes the peripheral clocks.

Bright-light exposure in the morning also leads to better alertness and less fatigue throughout the day and falling asleep earlier at night. This is because when we get sunlight in the morning, the SCN signals the body to reduce melatonin production, which helps us feel awake and alert during the day. At the same time, it helps boost and optimize cortisol production early in the day, which is when we want cortisol to be highest.

Remember how we discussed in "Understanding the Nervous System" that cortisol production follows a circadian pattern, peaking shortly after waking and gradually decreasing throughout the day, reaching its lowest levels at night (see page 27)? Disruptions to this pattern lead to multiple symptoms like daytime fatigue and difficulty falling asleep at night. By exposing our eyes to bright light in the morning, we can help support the optimal production of cortisol through the HPA axis, ensuring our circadian rhythm stays in sync. One study found that exposure to bright light in the early morning not only suppressed melatonin secretion but also triggered a significant (>50 percent) and immediate increase in cortisol levels.[5]

Exposing your eyes to morning sunlight is helpful no matter what but is especially important if you often wake up exhausted or if you scored high on the low cortisol questionnaire on page 49, as it can literally help boost your cortisol levels after waking. And if you scored high on the high cortisol questionnaire on page 47, don't worry—it won't push your cortisol too high but rather help regulate your natural rhythm.

One of my online students, Fionna, recently shared how this simple change in her morning routine has made a big difference in her sleep and energy levels. Fionna used to wake up feeling completely drained, and it would take a couple of hours (and a lot of caffeine) before she could function. Her usual routine involved dragging herself out of bed, rushing to get the kids ready, and grabbing a strong cup of coffee just to get through it all. But she decided to try something different. Instead of diving straight into the chaos, she started waking up 15 minutes earlier, giving herself a bit of quiet time before the kids woke up. She'd brush her teeth, make a cup of warm water with lemon, and step out onto her balcony. Living in a high-rise building with a view of the sunrise, she would spend about 10 minutes enjoying her warm drink and taking in the beautiful view. The change was subtle at first, but over time, Fionna noticed that she started sleeping better at night, waking up more easily in the morning, and feeling more alert and energized right after waking up.

To reap the benefits of morning light exposure, just like Fionna, try the following:

- Aim to step outside for a few minutes as soon as you can after waking up, ideally within the first hour. This can be as simple as spending a few minutes in your courtyard or garden, or even just opening a window or door and standing near it to soak in as much natural light as possible. It doesn't matter whether it's sunny or overcast; the key is to get outside rather than staying indoors. For context, on a sunny day, you may be exposed to up to 100,000 lux in direct sunlight and around 10,000–25,000 lux in shaded daylight. On an overcast day, light levels typically drop to around 1,000 lux, and on a rainy or very cloudy day, it's still usually above 500 lux. In comparison, typical indoor lighting ranges from just 100 to 300 lux.

- When natural light isn't accessible (such as in winter when the days are shorter or if you have to start work before sunrise), a bright light therapy device (often referred to as a light box or SAD lamp) for morning light exposure can be effective in managing circadian timing disruptions.[6]

LIMIT EVENING LIGHT EXPOSURE

As we've seen, exposure to artificial light sources has become pervasive, particularly during the evening hours. Not only do we spend less time outdoors during the day, but we also find ourselves exposed to multiple sources of artificial lighting after dusk. This can be a challenge for our circadian rhythms. When we expose our eyes to bright light in the evening, it suppresses melatonin production and makes it harder to fall asleep and stay asleep.

While it's not realistic to return to the dark evenings and nights of our ancestors, there are steps you can take to minimize the impact of light in the evening:

- Dim the lights in your home 1.5–2 hours before bedtime by using dimmer switches or lamps rather than relying on bright overhead lights. This gradual reduction in light intensity signals to your body that it's time to wind down and prepare for sleep. You can also get red or amber bulbs for your lamps, since those colors minimize the disruption of melatonin production, promoting better sleep quality.

- Limit blue light from electronic devices in the evening by refraining from using electronic devices such as smartphones, tablets, and computers at least 1 hour before bedtime. Alternatively, limit blue light from these devices using apps that filter blue light or built-in features on your devices to adjust the color temperature of the screen.
- After the sun goes down, consider wearing glasses that are designed to filter out the blue light emitted by electronic devices and artificial lights. These are called "blue-light-blocking glasses" and they have amber- or orange-tinted lenses, which filter out blue light.

ENSURE YOUR BEDROOM IS PITCH-BLACK

Darkness serves as a natural signal to the body, indicating that it's time to rest and prompting the release of melatonin. Any light exposure, even from dim sources like alarm clocks or ambient light from outside, can disrupt sleep stages and diminish overall sleep quality. These interruptions can lead to more frequent waking throughout the night, disrupting the body's natural rhythm.

To keep your bedroom as dark as possible at night, consider the following:

- Install curtains or blinds that block out external light sources, such as streetlights or car headlights, to create a darker sleep environment.

- Cover or dim any electronic devices in the bedroom, such as alarm clocks.
- Wear an eye mask if you can't control external light sources.

What practical steps can you take this week to better manage your light exposure? Can you make a habit of stepping outside or sitting near an open window for a few minutes as soon as you wake up? How about avoiding your phone before bed to reduce blue light exposure? Or, if your bedroom has too much light, maybe try sleeping with an eye mask. Remember, it's the small, consistent steps that lead to meaningful shifts.

Once you have mastered light exposure, let's move on to the next timekeeper—mealtimes.

Eat In Tune with Your Rhythm

We looked at eating consistently at the right times in Step Two, so hopefully this habit is already one you have integrated in your day. But along with balancing blood sugar, it is one of the most effective ways to synchronize the peripheral clocks, especially the ones in the gut, to optimize nutrient absorption and improve energy production.

Our bodies have evolved to anticipate and respond to regular mealtimes, and drastically changing the timing of food intake can impact our metabolic health. Animal studies have shown that altering feeding times disrupts synchrony within peripheral clocks, even when the SCN remains aligned with day–night cycles.[7] This desynchronization disrupts metabolic functions, potentially leading to long-term issues like obesity and insulin resistance.

Notice how you often feel hungry at around the same time each morning. This is your circadian rhythm at work. In anticipation of your usual breakfast time, your brain signals the release of ghrelin to stimulate appetite, your pancreas starts producing insulin to manage blood sugar levels, and your gut prepares digestive juices, all getting your body ready for the meal ahead.

However, erratic eating habits, such as skipping breakfast one day and eating it the next, can confuse your body's internal clocks. While your digestive system will still work to process food, eating at irregular times can disrupt its optimal functioning, leading to poorer digestion, greater blood sugar fluctuations, and reduced nutrient absorption.

Interestingly, eating breakfast (as opposed to skipping it, which was one of the habits we explored in Step Two) plays a significant role in regulating circadian rhythms and optimizing digestion, nutrient absorption, and blood sugar regulation.

Hopefully, you have now adopted the meal schedule outlined in Step Two (see page 134) to help you maintain consistency throughout the day. Now, let's look at some habits that will help you to build on this and align your food intake with your circadian rhythm, therefore maximizing your metabolic health, energy levels, and overall well-being.

EAT EARLIER IN THE DAY

Instead of eating most of your calories in the evening with a large dinner, try spreading them out by having bigger breakfasts and lunches. If you're used to eating small lunches or maybe just having a snack for lunch, this can feel a bit challenging at first, especially if you work in an office with limited time to eat. One simple solution is to cook extra dinner so you always have leftovers for lunch the next day. By eating more at breakfast and lunch, you'll avoid needing a large dinner. This approach works because our bodies process glucose and maintain insulin sensitivity better in the morning and early afternoon and worse in the evening and at night. By avoiding large meals at dinner, you'll be supporting your body's natural rhythms.

LIMIT YOUR EATING WINDOW TO 12 HOURS DURING THE DAY

Limiting your eating to a 12-hour window is a gentle form of Time-Restricted Eating (TRE), a practice that involves eating all your meals within a defined timeframe each day. For example, if you have breakfast at 8 a.m., aim to finish your last meal by 8 p.m. This aligns your eating schedule with the hours when your gut is naturally better equipped to process food (with more digestive juices, better blood sugar control, and improved nutrient absorption). It also gives your gut a break at night, when it's less prepared to handle food, and provides plenty of time for essential "housekeeping" tasks, such as the migrating motor complex, which clears waste and prepares the gut for the next day.

EAT AT ROUGHLY THE SAME TIME EVERY DAY, EVEN ON WEEKENDS

This is the power of anticipation that I mentioned earlier. When you consistently eat meals (and snacks) at the same times, your peripheral clocks start gearing up in preparation for the upcoming meal, optimizing their functions to efficiently process and utilize nutrients. Frequently changing your mealtimes or snacking at irregular hours may lead to inconsistencies in hormone secretion, digestive enzyme activity, and metabolic processes that can affect digestion and metabolic functions.

DRINK THE RIGHT BEVERAGES AT THE RIGHT TIME

To optimize the effects of drinks containing caffeine, such as coffee, green tea (including matcha), black tea, white tea, and yerba maté (and be mindful of other "hidden" sources like cocoa-based drinks, energy drinks, and sodas), it's best to drink them in the morning or early afternoon to avoid disrupting sleep later in the day.

Herbal teas, which are caffeine-free, can be enjoyed any time of the day and are great in the evening or before bed. These teas often contain calming ingredients like chamomile or lavender that promote relaxation and sleep. Examples of herbal teas that can be beneficial in the evening or at night are chamomile, lemon balm, and holy basil (tulsi). These teas can help the body and mind wind down, making them ideal choices for evening relaxation (see box below).

Calming Teas

CHAMOMILE TEA

Chamomile contains apigenin, an antioxidant that binds to certain receptors in your brain that may promote sleepiness and reduce insomnia.[8] Drinking a cup of chamomile tea 1 hour before bed can be a great nighttime ritual to promote relaxation and a good night's sleep.

Brewing instructions: Put 1 tablespoon loose-leaf tea into your strainer of choice. Steep in 1 cup boiling water for 5–10 minutes. Remove the strainer and enjoy.

Precautions: People with allergies to members of the *Asteraceae* family should exercise caution with chamomile. Chamomile may interact with certain medications, including blood thinners and sedatives, so consult a healthcare provider if you're on these or have underlying health conditions. Pregnant and breastfeeding women should use chamomile cautiously, as there is limited information on its safety.

LEMON BALM

Lemon balm or melissa has traditionally been used as a gentle nervine that can alleviate feelings of nervousness, tension, and anxiety. A systematic review and meta-analysis showed that lemon balm can improve symptoms of depression and anxiety.[9]

Brewing instructions: Put 1 tablespoon loose-leaf tea into your strainer of choice. Steep in 1 cup boiling water for 5–10 minutes. Remove the strainer and enjoy.

Precautions: Lemon balm may change thyroid function, reduce thyroid hormone levels, and interfere with thyroid hormone replacement therapy. Avoid lemon balm in states of hypothyroidism. Pregnant and breastfeeding women should use lemon balm cautiously, as there is limited information on its safety.

PASSIONFLOWER TEA

Passionflower is a botanical remedy that has traditionally been used to improve sleep quality and promote relaxation. Early studies suggest that it boosts the level of GABA (the main calming [inhibitory] neurotransmitter) in your brain.[10] This can result in relaxation, enhanced mood, better sleep, and pain relief.

Brewing instructions: Put 1 tablespoon loose-leaf tea into your strainer of choice. Steep in 1 cup boiling water for 5–10 minutes. Remove the strainer and enjoy.

Precautions: Do not use passionflower with older antidepressants called monoamine oxidase inhibitors. It might interact with other medications, including sedatives and blood thinners, so consult a healthcare provider if you're on such medications or have underlying health conditions. Avoid if pregnant.

What steps can you take to eat in tune with your circadian rhythm? Remember, introducing new habits will take a little bit of effort at first, so it's important to focus on small, achievable changes that will build over time. It all adds up, and soon you'll start to see the benefits of reinforcing your circadian rhythm—better digestion, improved sleep, steadier energy, and greater resilience to daily stressors. And the best part? As you experience these benefits, they reinforce the habits and make them easier to maintain.

Let's quickly revisit how habits form with an example of a habit you can introduce from this section:

- Cue (trigger): It's lunchtime.
- Habit (new behavior): You eat a larger, balanced meal using leftovers instead of just having a few crackers and hummus.
- Reward: Fewer cravings in the afternoon and less hunger, leading to a lighter dinner and better sleep at night.

A note for shift workers

I recognize that many of the strategies I have discussed so far may not be possible for you. Let me share a few tips now that can help minimize the disruptive effects of shift work on your circadian rhythm:

- **Avoid frequent rotating shifts:** If possible, try to avoid rotating shifts where you switch between day and night shifts often. The constant change in your schedule makes it harder for your body to adapt. If rotating shifts are unavoidable, try to negotiate a schedule where the changes are less frequent, giving your body enough time to adjust to each shift before switching again.

- **Prioritize early shifts over night shifts:** Early-morning shifts are far easier on your circadian rhythm than night shifts. If you have the option, try to work earlier shifts (for example, 5 a.m. to 1 p.m.) rather than starting at night.

Night shifts (for example, 11 p.m. to 7 a.m.) are the most disruptive to your circadian rhythm. If night shifts are unavoidable, there are some strategies you can adopt to reduce their impact:

- **Reduce light exposure:** As you near the end of your shift, reduce your exposure to light. Blue-light-blocking glasses can help with this.
- **Avoid sunlight on your way home:** Use dark sunglasses to block sunlight and go straight to bed once you get home.
- **Create a dark sleep environment:** Use blackout curtains or an eye mask to ensure your bedroom is as dark as possible.
- **Get sunlight upon waking:** After waking up, try to expose yourself to natural sunlight, or use a light box to simulate daylight before your shift.
- **Caffeine:** Consume caffeine in moderation, and avoid it at least 6 hours before the end of your shift.
- **Meal timing:** Eat a meal within an hour of waking, then schedule meals every 3–5 hours until you go to bed. For example, if you wake up at 4 p.m., eat before 5 p.m., then have a meal before your shift (around 9 or 10 p.m.), a snack during your shift (around 1 or 2 a.m.), and another meal a couple of hours before your shift ends (around 5 a.m.).
- **Avoid large meals before your shift ends.** Heavy meals may affect digestion and disrupt your sleep.
- **Bring healthy meals from home:** Preparing meals in advance ensures you're eating nourishing, balanced foods during your shift.
- **Stay hydrated:** Drink enough water, but reduce your intake a couple of hours before the end of your shift to avoid waking up while you sleep to go to the bathroom.

Now, let's shift our focus once more to physical activity.

Time Your Physical Activity

We looked at how movement can help you achieve better blood sugar control in Step Two, so hopefully you are already in the habit of spending 10 minutes moving your body after your main meals. In this step, we're going to build on that and see how exercise supports the body's internal clock, preventing disruptions in sleep and circadian rhythms.

It is well-known that engaging in regular exercise is linked to many health benefits, including cardiovascular health, weight management, muscle strength and bone density, and better sleep and mood. Interestingly, the timing of exercise can also influence circadian genes. Like light and food, exercise can help reinforce entrainment.[11] We will look at exercise in detail in the next step, but here I want to specifically talk about how to optimize the timing of movement to support your circadian rhythm.

Just like the best time to eat, the best time to exercise is during daylight hours and not too close to bedtime.

EXERCISE IN THE MORNING OR AFTERNOON

To promote optimal circadian rhythm, first try to avoid spending too many hours sitting down and being completely inactive during the day. If you have an office job that requires you to sit at your desk for most of the day, make sure you stand up and move your body regularly. Set a reminder to get up every hour for a few minutes—walk around, stretch, or do some light movement. If possible, take phone calls while standing or walking, use a standing desk, or walk to a colleague's desk instead of sending a message. A short walk after lunch, as you learned to do in Step Two, can be an excellent way to add a bit of movement into your working day.

When it comes to exercise, it doesn't really matter if you do it in the morning, afternoon, or early evening—the main thing here is to find a time that will be easy for you to stick with and try to maintain a consistent routine each week. This not only helps make the exercise habit stick (by reinforcing the cue, such as going for a walk after breakfast or lifting weights after work), but studies also suggest that exercising at more or less the same time can improve exercise performance. This is likely due to the body's muscle clocks, which adapt to regular training at specific times.[12]

Exercising in the morning, especially outdoors, is a great way of reinforcing two important timekeeping signals at once: light exposure and physical activity! Morning workouts also increase endorphin levels, which improve your mood, setting a positive tone for the rest of the day. I also love that completing your workout in the morning minimizes the risk of you missing it because of work, social obligations, or fatigue later in the day.

Exercising in the afternoon or after work also has its benefits. During this time, muscle strength and flexibility are typically at their peak, allowing for more effective workouts. Afternoon workouts can also help relieve stress accumulated throughout the day, improving mood and mental well-being.

While exercise has so many benefits, steer clear of intense workouts too close to bedtime. Engaging in vigorous exercise like going for a long run, doing high-intensity interval training (HIIT), or lifting heavy weights before bed can impact sleep quality. These types of exercises can elevate cortisol levels and delay the release of melatonin,[13] and they can raise body temperature and heart rate, making it harder for the body to wind down and prepare for sleep.

Instead, if you want to exercise after dinner, opt for an evening walk, a restorative yoga session, or gentle stretching. These gentler forms of exercise still provide benefits without interfering with sleep patterns.

Are there any ways you can adapt your daily exercise so your physical activity aligns with your circadian rhythm? What tweaks can you make this week? Can you get off the train or tram one stop earlier to fit in more walking in the morning? Or can you cycle to work or the school drop-off? If you have an office job, can you make a conscious effort to move more during the day using some of the tips provided? If you usually work out after dinner, will switching to a gentler form of exercise help prevent it from interfering with your sleep? And can you shift more intense workouts to the morning before work instead? These are just suggestions—find what works for you and your lifestyle. The key, as always, is consistency.

Fix Your Sleep

Getting "a good night's sleep" not only makes you feel great, but it's essential for mental and physical health. It improves your mood and cognitive function, optimizes digestion and blood sugar management, helps your body repair, and maintains all your systems working properly. So, getting enough restorative sleep is foundational for overall health and is one of the most important ways to increase your resilience to stress.

Sleep deprivation, on the other hand, is linked to increased blood pressure, higher evening cortisol levels, disrupted appetite, high insulin levels, high inflammation, and weakening immune function, as well as contributing to metabolic issues, insulin resistance, and weight gain, all worsened by circadian rhythm disruption. Additionally, sleep loss impairs cognitive function and contributes to emotional instability and mood disorders.[14]

It is clear that prioritizing sleep is one of the most important things you can do for your health. The steps you've already taken to synchronize your circadian rhythms, such as light exposure, meal timing, and exercise, will automatically support better sleep, but below are a few additional habits to help improve your sleep quality.

GO TO BED AND WAKE UP AT ROUGHLY THE SAME TIME (EVEN ON THE WEEKENDS!)

I know it's tempting to have a lie-in on weekends, but waking up and going to bed at approximately the same time each day (within a 30-minute window) is a simple way to improve sleep duration and quality. Just as with meal timing, our bodies thrive on consistency. When we establish a regular sleep schedule, our body begins to anticipate sleep and wake times, optimizing the production and secretion of melatonin and cortisol, which are key hormones involved in regulating sleep and wakefulness.

Start by choosing a wake-up time and bedtime that fit your lifestyle—let's say 7:00 a.m. wake-up and 10:30 p.m. bedtime. Set your alarm for 7:00 a.m. and stick to it, even on weekends. A sunrise alarm clock can help with this, as it gradually brightens to mimic natural sunlight, making waking up feel more natural and less jarring. Over time, your body will adjust, and you may no longer need an alarm. If you stay up later than usual one night, try to wake up at your usual time the next morning instead of sleeping in. This helps maintain your rhythm, making it easier to fall asleep at your regular bedtime the following night.

(A note for parents with babies or young children: If your nights are broken, don't stress about a perfect sleep schedule. Prioritize rest whenever you can, sleep in if needed, and focus on supporting your circadian rhythm in all the other ways discussed in this step.)

AVOID DAYTIME NAPS

While short naps can be beneficial for some people, excessive or long naps during the day can disrupt the sleep–wake cycle and make it harder to fall asleep at night. If you need to nap, aim for a short nap of no longer than 20–30 minutes early in the afternoon.

LIMIT CAFFEINE INTAKE AFTER MIDDAY

Caffeine is a stimulant that blocks adenosine receptors in the brain. Adenosine is a neurotransmitter that accumulates in the brain throughout the day, gradually increasing drowsiness and promoting sleep as the day progresses. By blocking adenosine receptors, caffeine counteracts these effects, leading to increased alertness and reduced feelings of fatigue. Try to consume caffeine only in the morning, because having it later in the day can make it harder to fall asleep and negatively impact the quality of your sleep.

AVOID HEAVY MEALS BEFORE BED

Eating large or rich meals before bed can cause discomfort or worsen reflux symptoms, making it harder to sleep. Additionally, eating heavy meals late in the evening can lead to blood sugar fluctuations, which may interfere with sleep quality. To promote better sleep, it's best to avoid large, heavy meals close to bedtime, and ideally try to have your last meal at least 2 hours before bed.

Also, be mindful of alcohol. While it may help you fall asleep initially, alcohol can disrupt your sleep later in the night, reducing sleep quality and leaving you feeling more tired the next day. Alcohol especially impacts one of the main sleep cycles called REM (rapid eye movement) sleep, which is crucial for cognitive function and memory consolidation.

TURN DOWN THE THERMOSTAT

Maintaining a cool temperature in the bedroom at night is key for promoting optimal sleep quality and supporting the body's natural circadian rhythm. The body's core temperature naturally decreases during sleep to facilitate restorative rest. Keeping the bedroom cool, typically under 70°F (21°C), helps to facilitate this temperature drop, signaling to the body that it's time to rest. This can be challenging, especially during the summer months. My tips here are to use lightweight cotton bedding and consider using a fan or air conditioner to circulate air. If budget is not an issue, you can explore investing in a temperature-controlled mattress cover.

CREATE A RELAXING BEDTIME ROUTINE

This could include activities such as reading a book, practicing relaxation exercises like deep breathing or meditation, or taking a bath. In fact, a hot bath or shower before bed can be particularly beneficial, as warming the skin dilates the blood vessels (known as peripheral vasodilation), and studies show that skin vasodilation, which promotes heat loss, can reduce the time it takes to fall asleep.[15]

Stick to the habits you have learned in this step as closely as possible, but remember, life can be unpredictable. You might have to travel across time zones or attend to unexpected responsibilities like caring for a sick child, and that's perfectly normal. Don't stress about those occasional disruptions. Instead, focus on following these habits as consistently as possible. By prioritizing your circadian health most of the time, you'll build resilience to handle occasional disruptions.

• • •

You have now completed Step Three: Regulate Your Circadian Rhythm. Supporting your circadian rhythm is one of the best ways to decrease allostatic load, improve the HPA axis, and make you more resilient to stress and disease. Now, return to the questionnaires on pages 47–50 and see if your scores have changed. Can you spot a downward trend in symptoms? Noticing even small improvements is a powerful way to track progress and stay motivated.

Key Habits to Incorporate in Step Three

Once again, I've included a checklist below to support you in making small weekly changes.

Week 5

Continue building on the habits you've established in the previous steps and start introducing some small changes to regulate your circadian rhythm progressively over the next 2 weeks.

☐ Expose your eyes to morning sunlight as soon as possible after waking up, ideally within the first hour. Step outside or open a window and stand by it for 10 minutes or, alternatively, go for a quick walk around the block.

☐ Dim the lights 1.5–2 hours before bedtime by using dimmer switches or lamps rather than relying on bright overhead lights.

☐ Limit exposure to blue light from electronic devices in the evening by avoiding smartphones, tablets, and computers at least 1 hour before bedtime.

☐ Keep a regular eating schedule. You should already have this habit from Step Two, but now also ensure your last meal is not too late—ideally, eat 2–3 hours before bed.

☐ Try to limit your eating window to roughly 12 hours during the day. For instance, if you have breakfast at 8 a.m., aim to finish your last meal by 8 p.m.

☐ Try drinking a relaxing cup of chamomile tea about 1 hour before bed.

Week 6

Continue with the habits from last week, such as getting natural light exposure in the morning and dimming the lights as nighttime approaches, and build on these with some new habits.

☐ Move your body throughout the day, but avoid strenuous exercise 1–2 hours before bedtime.

☐ Avoid heavy meals close to bedtime.

☐ Limit caffeine intake after midday.

☐ Keep your room dark and cool by using an eye mask if necessary and adjusting your thermostat or using a fan in the summer.

☐ Maintain a consistent sleep schedule by going to bed and waking up at roughly the same time every day, including weekends.

- ☐ Establish a relaxing bedtime routine, such as reading a book, practicing deep breathing, meditating, or taking a warm bath.

When you feel confident with the habits you've acquired in this step, proceed to Step Four, where we will dive into how to embrace exercise for optimal health and resilience.

Step Four

Exercise for Mind and Body Health

If you are in a bad mood, go for a walk. If you are still in a bad mood, go for another walk.

—HIPPOCRATES

You've worked really hard over the last few weeks integrating new habits that reduce hidden physical stressors while also strengthening your resilience to unavoidable sources of stress. In other words, you're expanding your stress bucket, building a stronger foundation for long-term health. You might have already noticed small shifts in how you feel, such as satiety after meals, fewer cravings, more stable moods, more energy, or better sleep at night. These changes may seem subtle now, but they're compounding beneath the surface. Let's take a moment now to celebrate all the little wins and acknowledge the progress you've made. Before diving into this next step, think about whether there are any areas where you need to spend a bit more time to really embed the new habits.

It's time now to delve into something we've touched on in both Steps Two and Three: moving your body. It's no secret that living an active lifestyle (versus a sedentary one) has remarkable health benefits. Regular exercise has been shown to reduce the risk of developing a wide range of conditions, including cardiovascular diseases, metabolic syndrome, cancer, anxiety, depression, and dementia.[1] This means that physical activity is *essential* for both your mind and your body. In fact, if exercise could be packaged into a pill, there's no doubt it would be the most prescribed, most effective, and least controversial medicine in the world!

Here's the interesting thing, though: Exercise is a stressor; it triggers a stress response in the body. However, it's what we call "good," or "hormetic," stress—a beneficial type of stress that helps us adapt better to future physical and psychological stressors. Exercise acts as a buffer against stress, helping the brain and body to adapt, recover, and become more resilient.[2] This happens in several ways, including regulating the stress response, changing brain regions like the hippocampus and prefrontal cortex (critical for emotional regulation and cognitive functions), reducing oxidative stress, and even switching on certain genes that improve stress adaptation over time.[3]

With all this in mind, I can't stress enough how important it is to keep going with the healthy habits you've already integrated and continue to include some form of exercise in your daily life. And, don't worry—if this is a habit you haven't yet adopted, it's never too late to start! However, I am well aware that many people find themselves frustrated by exercise. Some struggle to find the time and motivation to do it.

Others feel disheartened by the lack of results. And for some, exercise just doesn't make them feel good—and it even *exacerbates* their symptoms. Perhaps this is you and it's one of the reasons you've struggled to add some movement in the previous steps.

Believe me, I know exactly what it's like to have a troubled relationship with exercise. As a kid, I was always active and loved playing all kinds of sports—from basketball and soccer, to tennis and gymnastics. It was a way for me to spend time with friends, challenge myself with competitions, and most importantly, have fun! But, as I got older, something changed. Exercise lost its joy and stopped feeling like play. Instead, it became a tool to control my body shape, maintain my weight, and even punish myself for overindulging. My problem wasn't lack of motivation; my issue was that I was using exercise as a coping mechanism that wasn't healthy at all.

At the gym, I pushed myself because I believed that my workouts were effective only if I was left feeling sore, breathless, and drenched in sweat. These intense workouts left me feeling energized and kept my body in shape for a while. However, over time, they became less and less effective. My long runs on the treadmill or intense HIIT sessions started to leave me feeling exhausted and moody, and they failed to prevent me from accumulating belly fat.

It wasn't until I scaled back and changed my relationship with exercise that it began delivering the results I was after: more energy, less anxiety, better mood, more muscle, and less body fat. More importantly, I started to enjoy it again. I hope this step helps you do the same.

Not Too Much, Not Too Little

Let's start by debunking four common exercise myths that I hear from so many of my clients and that often lead to frustration and poor results:

1. **Intense cardio will make you "skinny":** Spending hours doing cardio isn't necessary to burn fat and achieve a lean, toned body. In fact, excessive cardio can raise cortisol levels too much, promoting fat storage.[4] Long workout sessions, such as endurance running or cycling, can lead to a more pronounced increase in cortisol levels compared to shorter, moderate-intensity workouts. This doesn't mean you shouldn't do cardio, though; you just need to find the right intensity and duration for you.
2. **Weight training will make you "bulky":** While this is typically not a concern for men, many women worry that lifting weights will make them too big or bulky. Unlike men, who have higher levels of testosterone that promote muscle growth, women have much lower levels, making it difficult to build a lot of muscle mass. In fact, for most women, weight training leads to a leaner, more toned body, not bulk. And beyond the looks, weight training improves metabolic health, enhances body composition, strengthens bones, and promotes overall longevity.
3. **The more you exercise, the better:** It's possible to have too much of a good thing! Excessive exercise can elevate cortisol levels, hampering muscle growth and fat loss and leaving you feeling drained and lethargic. One of the best ways to control cortisol is to shorten your training sessions and leave enough time for recovery.

4. **Everybody can do any type of training:** Some people, especially those who are already under a lot of stress, may need to carefully consider the form of exercise they engage in or at least decrease the intensity at first. This is especially true for those who feel completely depleted (not energized) after a workout, have difficulty recovering, and struggle with building muscle and losing fat. If you scored high on the low cortisol questionnaire on page 49, this might be you.

Take my client Linda, a 43-year-old mother of three and a partner at a busy law firm. Each morning, before her kids woke up, she used to go for a long run. She thought that the longer the run, the more calories she would burn and the easier it would be to lose the extra weight she had accumulated over the last few years. But despite her dedication, nothing seemed to work. She loved running and felt great while doing it, but afterward, she was completely drained for the rest of the day. And no matter how much effort she put in, that stubborn belly fat wouldn't budge. She was surprised to learn that long cardio sessions could exacerbate her already high stress levels, elevate her cortisol levels, and promote fat storage.

Determined to make some changes, we tweaked her exercise routine, trading her long daily runs for shorter, alternate-day sessions. We complemented these with weight lifting sessions at her local gym twice a week. Two months later, she told me, "I feel strong. While the scale hasn't shifted much, I've gone a size down, lost belly fat, and no longer feel constantly fatigued." For me, this is true success.

I wanted to share my story as well as Linda's because, while it's well-known that a sedentary lifestyle can be detrimental to our health, we often talk less about the other end of the spectrum—the overachievers who push themselves too hard. If you're dealing with a lot of stress and allostatic load, exercising too much could actually be making the problem worse instead of improving it. Moderation is then key. We need to find the sweet spot. It's also important to note here that, in some cases, excessive exercise is a part of a broader pattern of disordered behaviors, such as bulimia, which are often driven by a desire to control body weight to manage emotional distress.

In my experience, the key to incorporating exercise into your day is to find the right type of exercise, with the right intensity, and also make sure you actually enjoy doing it! This is how you reap the benefits of exercise in the long term, making it a beneficial stressor that makes you stronger and more resilient rather than a toxic stressor that pushes you further toward allostatic load.

Avoid a sedentary lifestyle and pushing yourself to the limit. Instead, find the sweet spot in the middle where moderation leads to success.

The generic advice of the US Department of Health and Human Services is for adults to do "at least 150 to 300 minutes a week of moderate-intensity, or 75 to 150 minutes a week of vigorous-intensity aerobic physical activity," ideally spread throughout the week. Adults should also do "muscle-strengthening activities of moderate or greater intensity that involve all major muscle groups on 2 or more days a week."[5] These guidelines align with those in the UK and Australia.

The aim of this chapter is to expand on this general advice and provide you with a more specific approach so you can harness the benefits of exercise in a way that's both efficient and safe. My goal is for you to rediscover your love of exercise. I want you to embrace it not merely as a calorie-burning tool but rather as a powerful (and very affordable) way of living a longer and more fulfilling life. Strong is the new skinny, and regardless of any past frustrations with exercise, you can achieve a strong body that will make you more resilient to stress.

If you have been exercising for years, this step will offer you insights into how to get the greatest benefits out of it. And if exercise isn't part of your routine (yet!), I hope it will motivate you to give it a shot, because even a little bit of daily activity is much better than no movement at all.

Find the Perfect Exercise and Intensity

You've probably come across two camps when it comes to exercise: those who swear by the incredible benefits of cardio and those who swear by the power of strength training. So, which one is actually right? The truth is that both are essential components of a well-rounded workout strategy. By blending activities that improve the heart and circulatory system (cardiovascular exercise) with those that boost muscle strength (resistance or strength training), you'll set yourself up for success.

CARDIOVASCULAR EXERCISE

Cardiovascular exercise involves activities that increase your heart rate and breathing for a sustained period. This type of exercise primarily targets the cardiovascular system, improving heart and lung function, increasing endurance, and burning calories. Typical cardio activities include walking, jogging, cycling, hiking, swimming, dancing, boxing, spinning, and other group classes. Engaging in cardio activities offers a plethora of benefits, including increased longevity and improved brain health.

According to a recent study, cardiorespiratory fitness is a powerful marker of longevity.[6] It has also been shown that endurance exercises like running, swimming, and hiking elevate levels of a protein known as brain-derived neurotrophic factor. Research indicates that this protein not only enhances memory and cognition, it also mitigates anxiety and depression in mice.[7] Similar effects may occur in humans. Studies also show that aerobic exercise leads to moderate to large reductions in depression scores when compared to antidepressants, based on a review of 11 RCTs.[8]

There are many types of cardiovascular exercises and different intensities, ranging from very light to very intense, often classified into five zones:

- **Zone 1:** Very light and easy activity. This could be a slow walk, warm-up, or cool-down. Your breathing is steady and it's easy to talk (50–60 percent of maximum heart rate).
- **Zone 2**: Light to moderate activity. Your breathing becomes a bit heavier, but you can still carry on a conversation, though it feels harder than Zone 1 (60–70 percent of maximum heart rate).
- **Zone 3:** Moderate to intense activity. Your breathing is noticeably harder, and holding a conversation becomes difficult (70–80 percent of maximum heart rate).
- **Zone 4:** Intense effort that challenges your body. Your breathing is fast, and you can only manage a few words

at a time. You can't sustain this pace for very long (80–90 percent of maximum heart rate).

- **Zone 5:** Maximum intensity, where your heart is working at its peak. You are out of breath and can't talk. You can only sustain this pace for a few seconds to a few minutes at most (90–100 percent of maximum heart rate).

Each heart rate zone offers different benefits and uses different fuel sources. Zones 1–2 primarily rely on fat for fuel, while Zones 3–5 predominantly use carbohydrates, with some protein breakdown at higher intensities. Zones 3–5 are best for improving cardiovascular fitness and increasing VO2 max (the maximum amount of oxygen your body can utilize during intense exercise), but higher-intensity training requires careful balance with recovery.

Recently, there has been a lot of interest in Zone 2, which is considered light- to moderate-intensity exercise. Zone 2 cardio hits a sweet spot that allows you to enjoy the perks of exercise without placing too much stress on your body and causes less fatigue. The beauty of exercising at this intensity level lies in its ability to provide fitness benefits without leaving you feeling completely drained or exhausted afterward. Doing most of your cardio exercise in Zone 2 will build a solid fitness foundation while minimizing the release of cortisol. This intensity can be especially beneficial if more intense exercise tends to leave you feeling "off." Does this mean that Zones 4–5 are not appropriate? Not at all—these zones can be very beneficial for some, but in small doses. If you're already quite fit and recover well, you might want to challenge yourself with exercise that allows you to get to Zones 4 and 5 (such as sprints/HIIT) to further boost cardiovascular fitness. Just be sure to keep the sessions short and follow them with adequate recovery.

Moderate activity, such as Zone 2 cardio, has been associated with reduced risks of heart disease, diabetes, and certain cancers.[9] Additionally, regular moderate exercise can improve metabolic health by enhancing the body's ability to use glucose and fat for energy, promoting metabolic flexibility, and increasing insulin sensitivity.

You can use two methods to determine if you are in Zone 2:

1. **Heart rate monitoring:** You can calculate your maximum heart rate (MHR) using the formula: 220 minus your age. Zone 2 typically falls between 60 and 70 percent of your MHR. For example, if you are 35 years old, your MHR is approximately 185. Zone 2 would then be 111–130 beats per minute.
2. **Talk test:** During Zone 2 cardio, you should be able to hold a conversation with some effort. This means you can talk in full sentences without getting out of breath, but you are exerting yourself enough that speaking requires some effort.

The recommendation by the Centers for Disease Control and Prevention and National Health Service is to do moderate aerobic activity (Zone 2) for at least 150 minutes per week, or 75 minutes per week of vigorous aerobic activity. Let's make this general advice more specific, because the optimal frequency and duration of cardiovascular exercise for *you* will depend on your current health, stress, and activity levels (please check with your doctor to make sure that starting a new exercise routine is appropriate for you):

- If you're just starting out, are feeling a lot of fatigue and exhaustion, or you scored highly for low cortisol on the questionnaire on page 49, start with *gentle* daily walks.
  - › To begin with, don't worry too much about hitting the right intensity. Even gentle walks are going to make your heart beat faster than at rest, and this is going to bring benefits to your cardiovascular system. The beauty of walking lies in its simplicity. It also allows you to adopt other practices from previous steps, like enjoying morning sun exposure (see page 150).
  - › Here's how to get started: Find a cue that triggers your walk. For example, this could be after breakfast, lunch, or work. Use that cue to consistently remind yourself to go for a walk. Over time, your brain will form new neural pathways, making the habit automatic. With repetition, walking will feel natural and require less conscious effort.
  - › Start with just 10 minutes and pay close attention to how you feel. If it feels good, gradually increase the duration or pace of your walks as your energy and fitness improve. Listen to your body and progress at a pace that works for you.
- As you become more comfortable, gradually extend the duration of your walks, but don't worry about the intensity yet. For example, you can extend to 30 or 40 minutes of walking a day. This can be done in one or more sessions—you could walk for 15 minutes in the morning and 15 in the evening, for example.

- As your form improves, start to increase your pace or tackle hills to reach Zones 2 or 3. Alternatively, you can now include other activities such as jogging, cycling, and swimming.
- Your goal is to eventually reach at least 150 minutes of moderate activity in Zone 2 per week (in separate sessions—for example, 5 sessions of 30 minutes each). This will establish a solid foundation of regular aerobic exercise.
- Once you have established this foundation, consider introducing more intense activities, such as going for a run or doing HIIT sessions (such as sprints). Note that when you do more intense exercise, you should keep your sessions shorter. For example, you might want to limit your run to 20 or 30 minutes or your HIIT session to 10 or 15 minutes, and make sure you leave plenty of time to recover. However, listen to your body. If you start feeling exhausted or burned out, notice weight gain or an impact on your sleep, it's essential to scale back.

Think about how you could introduce more cardio into your weekly routine using habit stacking, building on the habits you've already established (see page 55). For example, if you already take a short walk after meals for better blood sugar balance, try extending it or picking up the pace to get your heart rate up. If you step outside for morning sunlight, why not turn it into a walk or even a bike ride to stack the benefits of sun exposure and exercise in one go?

STRENGTH TRAINING

Strength or resistance training involves activities aimed at building muscle mass and improving muscle strength, endurance, and power. This type of exercise uses resistance to challenge your muscles. Examples include lifting weights, using resistance bands, or doing bodyweight exercises (such as push-ups, squats and lunges, pull-ups and planks). By consistently incorporating these exercises, your muscles adapt and grow stronger over time.

For many, the goal of strength training is to achieve a lean and athletic body, but that's just a bonus! Beyond improving body composition, having adequate muscle mass is linked to better overall health, increased longevity, and a higher quality of life:

- **Metabolic health:** Muscle tissue is a key player in maintaining metabolic health by regulating blood sugar levels and enhancing insulin sensitivity, which reduces the risk of type 2 diabetes. In one study published in the *Journal of Diabetes Research,* those who didn't do any strength training were 2.4 times more likely to have insulin resistance compared to those who did strength training for 1–2 hours a week.[10]
- **Bone density:** Strength training exerts mechanical stress on bones, stimulating them to become denser and stronger. This is crucial for preventing osteoporosis and reducing the risk of fractures, especially as we age. By engaging in regular strength training, you can enhance bone mineral density and maintain skeletal health.
- **Longevity:** Research has demonstrated a correlation between muscle mass and decreased all-cause mortality.[11] Maintaining adequate muscle mass through strength training is associated with a longer lifespan and improved overall health outcomes.

Unfortunately, our muscle mass and strength start to decline from as early as our thirties, and we lose muscle at a much quicker rate if we lead a sedentary lifestyle. This means that we need to be proactive and mindful of this muscle loss that happens with age. The more effort you're willing to put in now, the more benefit you'll reap in the future, and it's never too late to start.

Let's get into the evidence-based strategies to build muscle mass and strength in a way that takes into account your current capabilities. You will need to focus on:

1. Optimizing nutrition by focusing on eating enough protein (see Step One, page 69). Protein provides the building blocks your body needs to build muscle.
2. Challenging your muscles to make them grow with strength training.

Health guidelines recommend doing strengthening activities that work all the major muscle groups at least 2 days a week. Again, let's look at what this might mean for you (remember to check with your doctor before you start a new exercise routine to make sure it is appropriate for you):

- If you scored high for low cortisol on the questionnaire on page 49 and exercise in general makes you feel exhausted, start with 1 or 2 weekly sessions of *gentle* strength training. Yoga can provide effective strengthening benefits while being mindful of your body's capacity and limitations. Yoga is also one of the most effective somatic (body-based) therapies to regulate the nervous system and decrease stress (we will discuss more about it in the next step). Once your symptoms improve, you can increase the intensity by incorporating Pilates into your routine, which uses bodyweight exercises or a machine called a reformer to build strength. As you feel more capable, you can progress to strength training with weights.

- For everybody else, I recommend strength training with weights and/or a resistance band. Bodyweight exercises can also be effective if they are challenging enough to fatigue the muscles to a point where you struggle to do 1 more rep. If you are new to this type of training, it can be useful to seek the help of a qualified personal trainer to learn how to do each exercise correctly and help you create an exercise routine. Correct form is the top priority with any exercise. There are also multiple apps that can get you started, but here are some general guidelines:

    › Start with 2 full-body workouts per week. Make sure they are not on consecutive days to allow for proper recovery. The recovery period is just as important as your workout session—this is because while your workout kicks off the muscle growth process, the actual muscle growth happens while you're recovering. Each session should take around 45 minutes, though the time may vary depending on how long it takes you to complete each exercise.

    › Just like with cardiovascular exercise, create a cue that links the behavior to a specific time and place to help establish the habit. For example, you could choose to do it every Tuesday and Friday after work at your local gym. Try to keep these times as consistent as possible to ensure the habit sticks.

- Choose compound exercises that target multiple muscle groups simultaneously, such as squats, deadlifts, lunges, push-ups, rows, and overhead presses. These exercises provide the most bang for your buck and maximize muscle recruitment.
- Aim for 1–3 sets of each exercise, performing 6–12 repetitions per set, ideally getting 1–3 repetitions away from failure during most workouts, to stimulate muscle growth and strength gains.
- Allow 45–60 seconds of rest between sets to ensure adequate recovery and performance during each set.
- Gradually increase the weight or resistance used for each exercise as you become stronger and more comfortable with the movements. This progressive overload is essential for continued muscle growth and strength gains.

Before we move on to the next section, I want to emphasize two key points:

1. **Any movement is better than no movement at all.** While I've provided guidelines to help you build an optimal workout routine that includes both cardio and strength training, remember that you must listen to your body first. For example, if all you can manage right now is a short 10-minute walk each day and 1 yoga session a week, that's still a fantastic start. As you begin to feel the benefits, it

will become easier to gradually add more activities. Exercise has a compounding effect: The more you do it, the stronger you become, the easier it gets, the more fun it is, and the more you'll naturally crave it.

2. **Consistency beats perfection, always.** It's far more important to do a little bit each day than to try to do a lot only every once in a while. Regular, consistent effort will always yield better results over time.

Fueling your workouts

My clients often ask me whether it's necessary to eat before they exercise. If you're engaging in morning workouts without eating breakfast or if you've gone 5 hours without eating before hitting the gym, you're effectively exercising in a fasted state. While there is evidence to support fasted workouts accelerating fat burning, conflicting research suggests there are potential drawbacks to exercising on an empty stomach. For instance, a study published in the *Journal of Physical Therapy Science* found that exercising following an overnight fast was more effective at reducing body fat compared to non-fasted exercise.[12] However, participants who exercised in a fasted state experienced increased cortisol levels, which can jeopardize weight-loss efforts and muscle gains. This is especially true for long and intense workouts.

To minimize stress and prevent cortisol spikes during your workout, I recommend that, if you are going to do moderate- to high-intensity exercise for more than 30 minutes, you should have a snack before exercising if you haven't had breakfast or if it's been more than 4 hours since your last meal. Carbs are the ideal source of energy here, so focus on carbohydrates with a little bit of protein. Eating a piece of whole-grain toast with peanut butter 30 minutes before your workout, for example, would be great, or have a smoothie made with a banana and a couple of tablespoons of whey protein powder and water. Carbs will provide the energy you need to fuel your workout.

Another question I'm asked is: Do I need to have a post-workout snack or meal? After your workout, your body undergoes processes to repair muscle tissue and replenish the glycogen stores that were depleted during exercise. Carbohydrates are important for replenishing glycogen, but protein is essential for muscle repair and growth.

If you're engaging in low- or moderate-intensity cardio (for less than 1 hour), yoga, or Pilates, it's not strictly necessary to eat immediately after your workout, provided you're maintaining a balanced diet and not skipping meals (see Steps One and Two).

If you're doing weight lifting, long-duration cardio (for longer than 1 hour), or high-intensity cardio like HIIT, you'll benefit from a post-workout snack. Eating a snack with carbs and protein has been shown to promote greater muscle growth and exercise performance in subsequent workouts. Always include carbohydrates alongside your protein, as they work together to increase glycogen storage rates. Pairing a source of protein such as chicken with a source of carbs such as root veggies like sweet potatoes is a great combination. Another excellent option is cottage cheese with fruit.

By providing your body with the nutrients it needs to perform and recover, you can maximize the benefits of your efforts in the gym.

Before we wrap up Step Four, let's touch on two important factors that are often overlooked when it comes to women and exercise, yet they can make a big difference in how effective your workouts are. The first is synchronizing your workouts with your menstrual cycle, and the second is making small adjustments as you approach menopause to get the most out of your exercise.

Synchronize Exercise with Your Menstrual Cycle

If you menstruate, you've probably noticed that some weeks your exercise routine feels easier, while other weeks it feels much harder, even if you're following the same routine, getting the same amount of sleep, and eating the same sort of meals. This is because hormonal fluctuations throughout the menstrual cycle can affect your performance and tolerance to stress. Depending on where you are in your cycle, exercise is more or less taxing on your body.[13]

Most exercise protocols and recommendations are the same for men and women, but they are often based on data from studies where women are significantly underrepresented.[14] As a result, women often follow exercise programs that don't take into account their unique hormonal fluctuations. While men experience constant hormone levels throughout the month, leading to stable exercise performance, women experience hormonal changes throughout the menstrual cycle, driven by fluctuations in estrogen and progesterone. These hormones have distinct effects on the body, influencing factors like endurance, muscle growth, and recovery.

So, it makes sense to adapt our workouts to these hormonal changes in order to minimize stress and optimize the effectiveness for your strength and stamina. When you understand what's happening in your body each week, you can make a few tweaks to your exercise routine so you start working smarter not harder. This is what syncing your exercise routine with your menstrual cycle is all about.

Many of my clients, despite having had periods for most of their lives, feel confused about the changes that happen throughout their cycle. If that sounds like you, let me break it down for you. I'll briefly explain how your menstrual cycle works, how estrogen and progesterone fluctuate throughout the cycle, how each impacts your body and exercise performance, and what changes you can make to your exercise routine each week to align with these hormonal shifts.

THE MENSTRUAL CYCLE

A typical menstrual cycle lasts around 28–32 days and can be divided into four phases: menstruation and follicular phase (before ovulation), ovulation and luteal phase (after ovulation).

Menstruation (estrogen and progesterone are low)

The first day of your period is the first day of your cycle. This phase can be as short as a couple of days or a whole week, but the average is about 5 days. Both your estrogen and progesterone are at their lowest levels, and you might experience cramps and discomfort, especially in the first few days.

Follicular phase (estrogen production increases as the phase progresses, while progesterone remains low)

On around day 5 or 6 of your cycle (you might still be bleeding, but your period is probably finishing by now), your ovaries gradually start ramping up their production of estrogen and you might start feeling more energized, motivated, and focused.

Ovulation (high estrogen)

Your estrogen levels continue to rise, and around the middle of your cycle, typically around day 14 (though it can vary from day 11 to day 21), estrogen production peaks. This peak triggers a surge of luteinizing hormone (LH) from the pituitary gland. The LH surge causes a follicle to rupture and release an egg into the fallopian tube (ovulation).

Estrogen is highest in this phase, and it plays a significant role in improving exercise performance. It is an anabolic hormone (it helps build muscle), it improves how your body stores glycogen (the energy in muscles), and it makes the body more efficient at burning fat for fuel. This allows your body to rely more on fat for energy, sparing glycogen to some extent and delaying fatigue, particularly during longer-duration exercise. Estrogen also helps lower lactate, which can improve endurance. (Lactate is a substance that's produced when your body breaks down carbohydrates for energy without enough oxygen, often during intense exercise. As lactate builds up, it makes you feel muscle burn or fatigue.)[15]

In this phase you usually have lots of energy and training feels easier.

Luteal phase (high progesterone)

After ovulation, the ruptured follicle becomes a structure known as the "corpus luteum," which produces progesterone. While estrogen levels dip briefly after ovulation, they begin to rise again during the luteal phase. However, progesterone levels are dominant in this phase. If a fertilized egg isn't implanted, progesterone levels fall and you shed the lining and are back to day 1.

In this phase, which lasts about 2 weeks, progesterone is high. Progesterone increases heart rate and breath rate, and it increases core temperature, potentially making physical activity feel more difficult, especially in hot environments. It is also harder to repair and grow muscle because progesterone is catabolic, meaning it promotes the breakdown of muscle tissue rather than building it.[16]

In this phase, exercise can feel more challenging, as it may seem like you have to put in extra effort to complete the same routine that felt easier in the first half of your cycle. This is the time to dial it back and slow down to avoid unnecessary stress.

HOW TO SYNC YOUR EXERCISE ROUTINE WITH YOUR CYCLE

Now that you understand what's happening throughout your cycle, let's make a few adjustments to your exercise routine to get the most of it and minimize stress:

- Start by monitoring your menstrual cycle. Make a note of the first day of your period on a calendar or in a tracking app. Once you get closer to the mid-cycle, start monitoring signs of ovulation. Track changes in cervical mucus (which becomes clearer and stretchier). You may also experience mild ovulation discomfort or twinges. If you want to pinpoint exactly when you ovulate, you can also track your basal body temperature (BBT). Use a digital thermometer that reads to two decimal places, and take your temperature at the same time each morning before getting out of bed. One to two days after ovulation, your BBT will usually rise by about 0.5 to 1.0°F, signaling that you've entered the luteal phase.

- During your follicular phase and ovulation, focus on cardiovascular and strength-training exercises, as recommended previously, but here is when you can push yourself a bit more if your body feels good and ready. Consider going on longer walks or jogs and increasing your pace. Challenge yourself with heavier weights during strength-training sessions or maybe more reps. If you feel like trying a new challenging class at the gym, this is the time to do it!

- After ovulation, pay extra attention to how you feel; you might have to dial things down a bit in terms of intensity. Continue doing cardiovascular exercises, but avoid pushing yourself to new limits. You might need to decrease duration or pace, especially during the last week of the luteal phase as you approach menstruation. When strength training, instead of aiming for personal bests, maintain or reduce the weights, reduce reps or sets, and allow plenty of time for recovery between sessions. If you're not feeling up to lifting weights as you approach your period, opt for yoga or Pilates during the last week of your cycle as a gentler alternative.
- When your period arrives, it's perfectly okay to take a couple of days off if needed. However, if you feel great, you don't necessarily need to rest: The right movement can often relieve cramps and release tension in your muscles. Contrary to what some might think, many women feel better and stronger during their period because hormone levels are at their lowest. That said, if you experience heavy periods or severe cramps, it might be more appropriate to take it easy. Always listen to your body and do what feels right for you.

Consider keeping a journal to get to know your body throughout your cycle. As you train through several cycles, pay attention to how your body responds to training during each phase so you can identify when you are strongest and when you need to rest more.

Optimize Exercise During Perimenopause and Menopause

Menopause marks the end of a woman's reproductive years, but it doesn't happen suddenly; it's a series of changes involving hormonal fluctuations that occur over the course of many years (known as perimenopause) and have significant effects on a woman's physiology. During perimenopause, common symptoms include irregular periods, sleep problems, fatigue, headaches, hot flashes and night sweats, mood swings, brain fog, anxiety, and depression.[17]

One of the most common complaints I hear from my clients as they approach menopause is that they struggle to build muscle and keep their weight under control, even though they haven't changed the way they eat or exercise. This will make sense once you understand what is driving these changes:

- In the years before menopause, estrogen levels fluctuate and ultimately decline. Estrogen plays a crucial role in regulating metabolism and fat distribution in the body. The decrease in estrogen levels can lead to a redistribution of fat from the hips and thighs to the abdomen, resulting in increased visceral fat (remember, this is fat surrounding internal organs), which is associated with higher health risks.

- Estrogen increases insulin sensitivity, so, as estrogen declines, we need more insulin to get glucose out of the bloodstream and into the cells. In other words, cells become less responsive to insulin's signals, making it harder for glucose to enter the cells. When insulin levels are consistently high because of increased insulin requirements, this can lead to hyperinsulinemia. High levels of insulin in the bloodstream can promote fat storage in adipose tissue.

- Age-related loss of muscle mass and strength accelerates during the perimenopausal period. This loss of muscle tissue can decrease overall energy expenditure and lower physical activity levels, making it more challenging to burn calories and maintain a healthy weight.

All this doesn't mean we're doomed! It's simply a new phase of life that requires adjustments. Just as women in their reproductive years benefit from syncing their exercise routines to their menstrual cycles, women entering menopause can also adapt their diet and exercise routines to their declining hormone levels. A higher-protein diet combined with more resistance training can keep you strong throughout perimenopause, menopause, and beyond.

Here are some key strategies to use:

- Optimize nutrition during perimenopause and menopause by focusing on increasing protein intake while being mindful of carbohydrate consumption (see Step One, pages 77–85). This isn't to say that women in this stage should avoid carbs, but because of increased carbohydrate sensitivity, they often do better by moderating their intake.

A study published in *BJOG* shows a strong link between perimenopause, protein intake, and weight management.[18] The researchers propose that increasing protein could prevent weight gain during perimenopause because of the "protein leverage effect," a phenomenon whereby the body regulates its food intake primarily based on the proportion of protein in the diet. When it is low, the body tends to increase overall food consumption to meet its protein requirements, potentially leading to excess energy intake and weight gain. Protein high in leucine can be especially beneficial for muscle growth during menopause. Leucine is an essential amino acid that plays a crucial role in stimulating muscle protein synthesis (muscle growth). Protein sources such as whey protein, dairy products, eggs, and meat are high in leucine and can be beneficial for promoting muscle growth and preserving muscle mass during menopause. Additionally, branched-chain amino acid supplements, which include leucine, may provide extra support for muscle synthesis, especially if dietary protein intake is insufficient.

- Strength train 3 or 4 days a week, prioritizing weight lifting to stimulate muscle mass growth, improve strength, and promote bone health. While cardiovascular exercise remains beneficial and necessary, weight-bearing activities become particularly crucial during menopause to counteract the muscle loss and weakness associated with ageing. If your current exercise routine leans heavily toward cardio, consider reducing cardio sessions and allocating that time to exercises that challenge your muscles to failure and fatigue. An example of a well-rounded routine could include strength training on 3 alternate days, ensuring you target all major muscle groups, paired with 40 minutes of brisk walking on each of the remaining days.

- Discuss the potential benefits of menopausal hormone therapy (MHT) or hormone replacement therapy (HRT) with your doctor. This can help alleviate common symptoms of perimenopause and menopause, and research shows that MHT/HRT can help postmenopausal women maintain or increase muscle mass, strength, and performance. However, combining MHT/HRT with exercise results in better outcomes for muscle mass and function than either MHT/HRT or exercise alone.[19]

• • •

Congratulations on completing Step Four of the Cortisol Reset Plan! I hope you're feeling excited and inspired to harness exercise as one of the most potent tools for increasing your stress resilience and improving your health and longevity.

My goal is that you will have discovered ways to integrate exercise into your routine with moderation and recovery in mind, to maximize the health benefits. If you're just starting out, remember that even a small amount of movement is better than no exercise at all. Meet yourself where you are in your journey and aim to gradually boost your exercise and physical activity levels over time.

I hope you now feel less intimidated by exercise and have a clear plan for approaching it at any stage of your life.

Key Habits to Incorporate in Step Four

Below is a checklist with suggestions for introducing small movement habits into your day. Even though I recommend spending 1 or 2 weeks on each step, that doesn't mean you'll have an optimal exercise routine fully in place within a fortnight. Instead, think of these 2 weeks as a time to plant seeds, building small habits that will grow over time. Exercise is about giving your body the time it needs to adapt and get stronger. Trust the process—results won't come overnight, but with consistency, you'll be amazed at what your body is capable of!

Week 7

Remember to keep up with the habits you've integrated from the previous steps. Please go at your own pace and revisit the checklists if you need some motivation. This week, we'll focus on integrating some gentle movement into your days.

☐ First of all, I want you to think about which type of cardio activity is right for you—perhaps it's walking, jogging, or swimming; or maybe it's cycling, hiking or dancing. If you prefer exercising in a group, can you find a local class that fits into your schedule? Whatever you choose, the key is that you enjoy doing it!

☐ If you're just starting out, begin by introducing 15–20-minute *gentle* daily walks. You could also try a light full-body workout this week (such as yoga or Pilates).

☐ If you're more familiar with exercise, aim for at least 150 minutes of moderate aerobic activity (Zone 2) this week. This can include 5 days of 30-minute sessions of brisk walking, swimming, or light jogging. Try to do at least 2 full-body strength-training sessions this week, too. Ideally, focus on weight training.

☐ Whether you are new to exercise or more experienced, remember to schedule rest days between strength-training sessions.

Week 8

This week, let's build on the progress you made last week. You can also now start thinking about how you can fuel your body before and after workouts and track your menstrual cycle, if applicable.

☐ Try progressing to a daily brisk 30–40-minute walk (Zone 2, moderate intensity), depending on how new you are to exercise.

☐ Incorporate a full-body workout twice a week—either continuing with yoga or Pilates, or weight training. Remember to have rest days between sessions.

☐ Avoid working out fasted if you are going to do moderate or intense exercise. Fuel your body with protein and carbohydrates before workouts, and consider replenishing your body with protein and carbs after high-intensity or long sessions of cardio or strength training.

☐ If applicable to you, track your menstrual cycle and start adjusting the intensity and duration of your exercise routine accordingly.

☐ If you're in perimenopause or menopause, focus more on strength training. A great routine could be 3 days of strength training, alternated with 30–40 minutes of brisk walking on the days you're not strength training.

You've integrated so many new habits over the last few weeks that have reset your cortisol levels, decreased physical stressors, and boosted your energy reserves. I hope you've started to notice a real difference in how you feel. Take a moment to revisit the questionnaires on pages 47–50 and assess how you're feeling after 2 more weeks of work. Remember, celebrate every win—no matter how big or small!

In the last step, we'll be addressing those perceived stressors we talked about in Part I. You might find that some resistance comes up as you work through this step, but with the physical stressors reduced and your energy reserves—your "budget"—replenishing, you have built the capacity and resilience you need to be able to tackle it much more successfully.

Step Five

Build Psychological Resilience and Well-Being

In the depth of winter, I finally learned that within me there lay an invincible summer.
—ALBERT CAMUS

So far, with the first four steps of the plan, you've tackled the most common physical stressors that often fly under the radar but significantly contribute to your allostatic load and drain your energy and capacity. By applying the simple habits discussed in each step, you've reduced these unnecessary stressors, freeing up energy that was being wasted and boosting your "stress bucket" capacity.

By reducing the activation of the stress response (and the prevalence of cortisol) and by conserving energy resources while incorporating habits that optimize mitochondrial function and energy production, you've been boosting your stress resilience. This helps you handle and adapt to stressors more effectively, minimizing the risk of maladaptations that could negatively impact your health. Now, let's shift our focus to *perceived* stressors rather than physical ones.

Remember, perceived stressors are psychological or emotional, and they can be real or imagined. Physical stressors are actual threats to homeostasis, while psychological and emotional stressors are anticipatory and not always based in reality. For example, you might say hello to someone you know, but they don't say hi back. Your brain might interpret this as them not liking you or being upset with you. But that doesn't mean it's true—they could have not heard you or they could have been distracted. The key characteristic of these stressors is that they can trigger the stress response, whether or not they are real threats.

Everyone reacts differently to these types of stressors, with some people having more tolerance and flexibility than others. Have you ever wondered why some people seem to handle challenges with relative ease, while others get easily overwhelmed by any setback? It's because their brain and nervous system have been wired and trained over time to respond in different ways. Where do you feel you are on this spectrum?

The way we interpret what's happening around us and how much control we feel we have over our environment are strongly influenced by many factors, including our genetic makeup, our current levels of stress, and past adverse experiences, particularly during childhood development. These interpretations and the reactions to them are not *conscious*, they are automatic "programmed" responses mediated by the ANS, operating below the level of our awareness.

During childhood, the connections between neurons (brain cells) are rapidly formed, strengthened, or reorganized. This heightened neuroplasticity allows children to learn new skills quickly, such as how to talk, walk, or write. However, it also makes their brains highly sensitive to environmental influences, both positive and negative. During this period, the brain is "programming" how we interpret and respond to the world, often becoming automatic patterns that persist into adulthood. Nurturing environments, where caregivers model self-regulation and healthy ways of managing challenges, help promote better emotional regulation and more flexible responses to stressors later in life. In contrast, adverse or traumatic experiences, as well as growing up in high-conflict homes or with caregivers who react to stress in less regulated ways (for example, yelling, constant arguing, or withdrawal), can lead to hypervigilance and a reduced ability to adapt to stress in adulthood.[1]

Traumatic experiences later in life can have similar effects.[2] Psychological trauma, whether from early life or later experiences, as well as high current stress levels can lead to changes in the brain and dysregulation of the nervous system. This dysregulation can make the nervous system overly sensitive to cues of danger, making it harder to stay in a regulated homeostatic state. It can also make the interpretation of sensory messages by the brain less accurate or "faulty," which reduces the ability to accurately assess and respond to the real demands of the environment, ultimately contributing to increased stress and more cortisol. Paradoxically, the very system designed to keep you safe (the nervous system) ends up contributing to your allostatic load.

When your body remains in a chronically activated state, as we've discussed before, you can think of it as being metabolically "expensive," consuming a lot of energy and resources to sustain. For optimal health, your body needs to remain in a lower-stress state most of the time. A dysregulated nervous system impairs your body's ability to heal and maintain long-term health.

The good news is, we're not doomed by our past experiences. Neuroplasticity is not something that happens only in childhood—the brain and nervous system can change and adapt at any point in our lives with enough practice and repetition. Just as you've been harnessing neuroplasticity by incorporating new habits in the first four steps, you also have the power to improve how your brain interprets the world around you, as well as how you respond and adapt to your environment.

In this step, we'll focus on increasing your nervous system flexibility and resilience through awareness, somatic (body-based) work, and brain training, to help you interpret threats better and respond to stressors in a more regulated way. As you improve your ability to self-regulate, you'll gain greater control over your environment and reduce the frequent activation of your stress response. This helps prevent your body from being constantly flooded with stress hormones like cortisol and can lower your allostatic load. When your nervous system is flexible, you can quickly reset and restore balance without lasting consequences.

The Six Building Blocks of Psychological Resilience

I have developed a framework for building resilience and psychological well-being that I use with my clients to support them in managing stress without becoming overwhelmed by it. The six building blocks of psychological resilience are:

1. **Awareness**, which helps you to understand and recognize your internal world of feelings, thoughts, and emotions.
2. **Connection to your body**, allowing you to tune into your physical sensations and regulate through somatic practices.
3. **Connection to Self**, based on the Internal Family Systems (IFS) model of therapy created by Dr. Richard C. Schwartz (see page 233), which integrates and balances the different parts of your psyche.
4. **Connection to others**, which focuses on the importance of positive interactions with others and safe, caring relationships.
5. **Time in nature**, which has a soothing effect on your nervous system and makes you feel part of something bigger.
6. **Finding your purpose**, which can guide you toward a sense of fulfillment and meaning in your life.

We'll go through each of these in turn, and I'll introduce practices to help you nurture your psychological well-being, build emotional resilience, and achieve a calmer, more balanced state.

The goal in this step isn't to *avoid* difficulty and distress (which is a normal part of life), but to develop the capacity to navigate life's challenges and recover from them more effectively, preventing lasting harm to your body and mind.

Build Awareness

To become better at regulating your nervous system, you need to *get to know* it and understand your internal world (feelings, sensations, and emotions), as well as your pattern of reactions and behaviors toward the world around you. This is achieved by becoming an *observer*. Most of your behaviors and reactions are automatic, but by bringing them into your conscious awareness, you establish the first step toward modifying ingrained patterns.

You are not an "anxious," "needy," or "too sensitive" person; your nervous system is just trying to keep you safe in the best way it knows how. The issue is that it might have learned responses that no longer serve you, and it could be misinterpreting signals of safety and danger, a process known as faulty "neuroception," which is contributing to your dysregulation. These are things that can be changed.

Dr. Stephen W. Porges, who developed polyvagal theory, coined the term *neuroception* to refer to our body's automatic (and unconscious) process of detecting and interpreting cues of safety or danger from both the external environment and inside the body. Neuroception interacts with our ANS to manage survival responses, influencing our emotional and physical states.[3]

As we touched on in "Understanding the Nervous System," neuroception is based on two main types of sensory input:

1. **Interoception:** our ability to sense internal bodily signals, such as feeling hungry, thirsty, changes in heart rate, breathing patterns, muscle tension, and pain.
2. **Exteroception:** our ability to sense the external environment through our five senses: sight, hearing, taste, smell, and touch. For example, it helps us detect a loud noise, recognize a friendly- or an angry-faced person, or feel the warmth of the sun on our skin.

The brain continuously interprets both interoceptive and exteroceptive inputs to assess whether we are in a state of safety or danger. Neuroception, using both interoception and exteroception, plays a crucial role in regulating the ANS and influencing our physiological, emotional, and behavioral responses to the environment.

Now, let's explore the three primary responses that the ANS can deploy, based on Dr. Porges's polyvagal theory. We will be calling these your three main *nervous system states.*

RELAXED (VENTRAL VAGAL)

This is the most comfortable state, which happens when our nervous system detects cues of safety. In this state, survival responses are inhibited. We feel calm, safe, and grounded, allowing us to think clearly and feel hopeful, inspired, and curious. It becomes easier to express ourselves and connect with others authentically. It's a highly social state, where caring for and helping others feels natural. If our nervous system detects cues of danger while in this state, we are more likely to seek connection and try to engage or cooperate with others to seek safety.

This state is also known as your "window of tolerance," a term coined by Dr. Daniel J. Siegel, a clinical professor of psychiatry at UCLA School of Medicine, that refers to the ideal "zone" where we function and thrive most effectively in daily life.[4] Beyond this "optimal zone" lie two other states: the hyperarousal zone (mobilized) and the hypo-arousal zone (immobilized).

Biological responses: Heart rate is normal, breathing is steady and deep, muscles are relaxed, digestion is functioning optimally, and the body is in a state of rest and repair.

MOBILIZED (SYMPATHETIC)

As the neuroception of danger increases, if seeking connection hasn't resolved the threat, the nervous system will switch from the ventral vagal state to the sympathetic state, also called the fight-or-flight response (see page 20 for a reminder of this).

Mobilization is crucial for responding to challenges, allowing you to either confront the threat head-on or run away from it. In this state, you may feel a surge of energy in your body, making it difficult to sit still. It is common to feel anxious, fearful, worried, or angry. This state is also called the hyperarousal zone.

Biological responses: Heart rate increases, breathing becomes fast and shallow, and muscles tense, preparing the body for action.

IMMOBILIZED (DORSAL VAGAL)

Finally, if fleeing or confronting the threat is not possible, or if the sympathetic response becomes too overwhelming, the body may shut down by shifting to the third state, the immobilized or dorsal vagal state. This state is characterized by energy conservation and numbing of physical and emotional sensations. In this state, we might feel hopeless, depressed, numb, and disconnected from our bodies. Social connections become difficult, and we tend to withdraw from others in this state. This state is also called the hypo-arousal zone.

Biological responses: Heart rate might be low to conserve energy, muscle tone is decreased, and the body may feel tired, numb, heavy, or disconnected.

There are also "hybrid" states, which combine elements of the three main states. For example, when playing sports or dancing with friends, you experience a mix of relaxed and sympathetic states, feeling calm but energized, ready to engage and take on challenges. Or when you are in a peaceful, reflective state like when you are meditating, you might experience a blend of relaxed and immobilized states. Or when you're caught between the urge to act and feeling stuck, it's a mix of mobilized and immobilized states, also known as the "freeze" state.

How to Cultivate Awareness

We naturally want to stay in the relaxed state (ventral vagal) as much as possible, but each response has a purpose and serves to protect us by adapting to the changing conditions of our environment. It is absolutely normal to experience all states, but the key is to avoid getting stuck in the survival states of mobilization or immobilization (as well as the hybrid state of freeze) and to be able to move flexibly in and out of these states, returning to our most healing state, the ventral vagal state, as quickly as possible.

Let's imagine a scenario where you've just had a heated argument with a friend about a sensitive topic that you are very passionate about and you can't seem to agree on. Your heart rate increases, your face feels hot and you speak faster and louder. As you walk away from the argument, you start to feel uneasy and keep replaying what you both said in your head over and over, and you start to worry that your relationship has been damaged. A few hours later, when you go to bed, you're still ruminating about what happened and find it difficult to fall asleep. Your nervous system is stuck in a survival state and is finding it hard to get back to a regulated, relaxed state needed to fall asleep.

To help bring regulation, you first need to bring *awareness* to what is happening inside your body. When you introduce awareness, you become attuned to your body's sensations, emotions, and feelings. You notice the messages that your body is sending you, such as shallow breathing and a racing heart, and you notice your persistent ruminating thoughts; this helps you identify your autonomic state ("I am mobilized or in a sympathetic state"). By doing so, you create a little space or pause that can help stop an automatic response/reaction (ruminating), and you can then choose a regulating practice instead (such as moving your body or doing a breathing exercise), which might be enough to shift you out of survival mode and back into a regulated state. While you may still feel unsettled, you no longer find yourself feeling overwhelmed.

To cultivate awareness, we will use three practices. The first will focus on improving your interoceptive accuracy so you can better listen to and understand what your body is trying to tell you. The last two will help you identify and recognize your nervous system states and the events that bring you in and out of each state.

It's important to note that awareness doesn't require you to change anything just yet. You will learn regulation practices in the following sections of this chapter, starting with somatic or bottom-up approaches using your body, followed by top-down approaches using your mind. For now, simply focus on bringing the unconscious into conscious awareness.

PRACTICE #1: INTEROCEPTION

As we discussed earlier, interoception is our ability to sense internal body signals like hunger, thirst, temperature, a racing heart, shallow breath, tension, or pain, providing continuous feedback to the brain of what is happening in the body. This information helps us understand the emotional messages our bodies are sending. Some messages, like butterflies in our stomach when we're excited, are easy to "hear," but others, such as a clenched jaw or shallow breathing when we're under stress, are subtler. Many of us might also be quite disconnected from bodily sensations, but this is something we can practice and improve. The more you listen to your body, the easier it becomes to interpret what it truly needs. By doing this, you'll start to influence your nervous system states and respond more effectively.

Here is a practice that will help you bring awareness to interoception:

1. Sit down and close your eyes. If closing your eyes doesn't feel comfortable, leave them open with a soft gaze, avoiding focusing on anything specific.
2. Begin by focusing on your breath. Don't try to change it; just observe whether it's fast or slow, shallow or deep.
3. Shift your attention to your posture. Are your shoulders tense or relaxed? Is your back straight or slouched?
4. What type of energy do you feel in your body? Do you feel restless and fidgety, calm and grounded, light and energized, or heavy and sluggish?
5. Shift your focus to the sensations in your body, particularly in your belly, chest, neck, and jaw. Do you notice any tightness or tension, or do these areas feel open and relaxed?

6. Make a practice of doing this daily so it becomes easier to tune in to the messages your body is sending.

If you feel overwhelmed during this exercise, especially if you're feeling activated and the body's signals are too intense (such as noticing a racing heart rate), open your eyes and focus on external cues in your environment. Focus on what you can see or hear around you, and notice the sensation of your feet on the ground or the chair you're sitting on. This will help ground you and bring a sense of calm.

PRACTICE #2: IDENTIFY YOUR NERVOUS SYSTEM STATES

The second practice to improve your awareness is to chart your nervous system states to be able to identify what state you are in at any given time.

Remember that there are three main autonomic states: relaxed (ventral vagal), mobilized (sympathetic), and immobilized (dorsal vagal). You are now going to embody each of these three states and take notes so you can articulate, as clearly as possible, the body sensations, thoughts, and emotions that accompany each state for you. The more details you can provide, the better. Print a blank sheet on my website via the QR code below or use the one on page 214. I've also included an example on page 215 so you can see what it might look like once you've completed the exercise.

Start with your *relaxed* state first:

1. Close your eyes or keep a soft gaze and think of a recent experience when you felt calm, grounded, and open. For instance, think about a leisurely walk in the park on a sunny day or catching up with a friend over a cozy cup of coffee. Try to replay the experience in your mind as vividly as possible, like watching a movie.
2. Now, shift your focus to the sensations in your body. Notice and describe them as fully as you can. Perhaps your breath is slow and deep, your shoulders relaxed, your body warm and at ease. How is your posture?
3. What type of energy do you feel? Do you feel calm and grounded?
4. Turn your attention to your thoughts and emotions. Describe them in as much detail as possible. Your thoughts may be neutral or positive, and your emotions might include contentment, optimism, gratitude, and confidence in your ability to handle any challenges that might arise.
5. Now, throughout the day, whenever you catch yourself in this state, shift your attention to your body sensations, thoughts, and emotions. See if you can identify or articulate any additional details you may have missed and update your chart. The more attuned you become to these cues, the easier it will be to recognize and deepen your awareness of this state.

Now, let's shift to the *mobilized* state:

1. Close your eyes or keep a soft gaze and think of a recent experience when you felt activated. Try not to think of

something too overwhelming; instead, look for something mildly activating. For example, you might recall a driver cutting you off in traffic or receiving a last-minute work email just as you were about to log off. Try to replay the experience in your mind as vividly as possible—again, like watching a movie.

2. Now, shift your focus to the sensations in your body. Notice and describe them as fully as you can. Perhaps your breath is shallow and fast, or maybe you are clenching your jaw and your shoulders feel tense. Do you feel a knot in your stomach? Does your chest feel tight? Has your heart rate increased?
3. What type of energy do you feel? You might feel alert and ready to tackle issues, but you might also be feeling a sense of urgency that is making you a bit on edge. Do you sense a surge of energy that is making you fidgety?
4. Turn your attention to your thoughts and emotions. Describe them in as much detail as possible. What thoughts are running through your mind? Are you being self-critical or judging others harshly in this state? What emotions are you experiencing? It could be frustration, irritation, anger, or anxiety, or perhaps a sense of urgency, impatience, or even overwhelm.
5. After you've fully articulated what this state feels like for you, try to release the activation taking a few deep belly breaths, with a longer exhale than inhale, and by focusing for a few minutes on your surroundings. What can you see? What sounds can you hear? Focus on the sensation of your chair beneath you, the feeling of your feet on the ground, or any other tactile sensations in your environment to help ground you back into the present moment.

Now, let's shift to the *immobilized* state:

1. Close your eyes or keep a soft gaze and think of a recent experience where you felt withdrawn or had a mild sense of hopelessness, something not too intense or overwhelming. For example, it could be a moment when you felt left out of a group conversation or when you faced a minor setback at work that made you question your abilities.
2. Now, shift your focus to the sensations in your body. Notice and describe them in whatever way that resonates for you. You might feel a heaviness in your body, a sense of numbness or disconnection from your body, or a lack of energy. There might also be a sensation of tightness or constriction in your throat or chest or a sinking feeling in your stomach.
3. What type of energy do you feel? Is your energy low or sluggish? Do you notice a sense of heaviness? Or does it feel scattered or drained, like you're running on empty?
4. Turn your attention to your thoughts and emotions. Describe them in as much detail as possible. What thoughts and beliefs are running through your mind? Are there pessimistic thoughts, doubts, or a sense of unworthiness? What emotions are you experiencing? It could be shame, loneliness, sadness, or feeling like you are broken or disconnected.
5. After you've fully articulated what this state feels like for you, it's a good idea to bring gentle movement to bring some energy back into your body. You could take a slow walk, do some gentle stretches or stand up and sway side to side to help bring your nervous system back to a more regulated state.

AUTONOMIC STATE	MY PHYSICAL SENSATIONS	MY THOUGHTS	MY EMOTIONS
Relaxed			
Mobilized			
Immobilized			

For example:

AUTONOMIC STATE	MY PHYSICAL SENSATIONS	MY THOUGHTS	MY EMOTIONS
Relaxed	• My breath is slow and deep. • There's a warm sensation throughout my body. • My heart rate is steady and calm. • My chest is open and my shoulders are relaxed. • My facial expressions feel soft and gentle.	• I'm focused on positive or neutral things. • I'm thinking about how to connect or engage with others. • My mind feels open and receptive to new ideas.	• I feel content. • I feel hopeful and optimistic about the future. • I'm grateful. • I feel connected to myself and others. • I can trust.
Mobilized	• My breathing is quick and shallow. • My muscles feel tense and tight. • My heart is racing. • My skin feels clammy or sweaty. • I'm fidgeting or restless. • My chest feels tight and my jaw is clenched. • There's a surge of heat or energy in my body.	• I'm focused on potential threats or problems. • I'm thinking about what needs to be done. • I'm trying to find quick solutions. • I'm being critical toward myself. • I'm being critical of others.	• I feel anxious or fearful. • I'm frustrated and irritated. • I'm angry. • I feel a sense of urgency.
Immobilized	• My breathing is slow or shallow. • My body feels heavy and sluggish. • My muscles are weak. • I feel numb. • My hands and feet are cold. • My posture is slumped. • I feel physically disconnected.	• My thoughts are self-defeating, such as "I can't do this." • I'm pessimistic about the future: "Things will never get better." • I'm struggling to think clearly.	• I feel hopeless. • I feel lonely. • I feel sad. • I feel isolated. • I have shame or guilt. • I feel indifferent, like I can't care or feel anything.

Once you've finished your chart, use it daily as a check-in tool. Frequently assess your current state by asking yourself, "What is my nervous system state right now?"

As you begin to observe your autonomic states throughout the day, you will start to notice that certain situations (places, people, events) have the tendency to shift you from your relaxed state into your survival states (we will call them triggers) and certain situations do the exact opposite (we will call them glimmers). Now, use the next practice to identify what those are.

PRACTICE #3: IDENTIFY YOUR TRIGGERS AND GLIMMERS

When our nervous system detects "triggers"—signs of danger—it activates the survival states of mobilization (sympathetic) or immobilization (dorsal vagal). On the other hand, when it perceives "glimmers"—a term introduced by Deb Dana, a trauma therapist specializing in the polyvagal theory[5]—the ANS shifts into the relaxed, ventral vagal state, promoting a sense of calm and connection.

Everyone's triggers and glimmers are different, but once you become aware of them, you'll be better prepared by anticipating the events that might push you into survival mode. This awareness allows you to make changes to avoid the trigger or introduce cues of safety that will help you return to a regulated state more quickly. For example, you might notice that congested traffic always shifts your nervous system into a mobilized/sympathetic state. With this knowledge, you can either change your route or departure time to avoid the trigger or introduce a cue of safety, like listening to calming music, humming, or taking deep breaths, to help you stay regulated.

Triggers: Triggers make us perceive danger so the ANS activates the state of sympathetic mobilization or dorsal vagal immobilization. Triggers could be people, places, or situations that create a sense of danger.
Glimmers: Glimmers foster a sense of safety, giving you the opportunity to relax into moments of connection with yourself, others, or the environment. Glimmers can cue our nervous system to stay in a calm and relaxed state or help bring back to regulation a nervous system that has shifted to survival mode.

Now it's time to create your triggers and glimmers list. Print a blank sheet from my website via the QR code below or use the one provided on page 218. Again, I have included some examples for you.

1. Start by identifying all the people, places, or events that instill a sense of danger and disrupt your feelings of safety, calm, and connection. These are your triggers.
2. Next, note the people, places, or events that instill a sense of safety, bring you calm and joy, and put a smile on your face. These are your glimmers.

MY TRIGGERS	MY GLIMMERS

For example:

MY TRIGGERS	MY GLIMMERS
• crowded places • loud noises • a difficult family member • a difficult boss or co-worker • being criticized or feeling judged • financial stress or unexpected expenses • watching the news • being ignored in a conversation • traffic • being late • social media • phone notifications	• taking a walk in nature • listening to my favorite music • watching a sunset or sunrise • engaging in creative activities like painting or writing • talking to my best friend • practicing mindfulness or meditation • enjoying a warm cup of tea or coffee in a cozy setting • being hugged or cuddled by a loved one • playing with my kids

Continuously refer to and update this list to gain a deeper understanding of the events that shift your nervous system states. Understanding what triggers a survival state and what brings you back to safety can give you a sense of more control over your environment.

Through these three practices you are cultivating the awareness you need to be able to listen to and understand the ongoing conversation between your body and mind. This new awareness empowers you to pause and change the automatic embedded responses that are contributing to your dysregulation. To integrate these practices into your daily routine, I recommend checking in with your body a few times a day, perhaps using a specific cue, like every time you drink a glass of water. Take a moment to breathe and tune in to the physical sensations you notice. See if you can identify your current autonomic state (whether you are in a relaxed, mobilized, or immobilized state), and see if you can pinpoint any triggers (for example, "my boss just sent me an email") or glimmers (for example, "I went for a relaxing walk around the park") that might have influenced it. At this stage, the goal is simply to get to know your nervous system better.

In a way, awareness is already a form of regulation (even without changing anything else) because it pulls your brain out of its automatic, predictive tendencies and brings you into the present moment. We are now going to build on that foundation by focusing on connecting to your body to regulate your nervous system.

Connect to Your Body

Let's move out of the survival nervous system states (mobilization and immobilization) and into our most healing state, the relaxed state, and we are going to do so by creating a sense of safety within our bodies using body-based or somatic exercises.

Building safety within your body means sending messages of safety from your body to your brain. We do this by engaging your body's natural regulation mechanisms, notably the vagus nerve, which is a key part of the PNS (see page 35 for a reminder of the crucial role the vagus nerve plays in regulation).

I am sure you have noticed that when you're dysregulated or feeling strong emotions, trying to "think your way out of it" (a top-down approach) is not very effective. This is because when we are under stress, the more primitive parts of our brain in charge of survival become more active, while activity in the prefrontal cortex (responsible for rational thinking and emotional regulation) decreases. As a result, the thinking brain becomes less effective at regulating emotions.

Instead, a more effective method is to focus on modifying physical sensations (a bottom-up approach). This doesn't rely on *thinking* but rather working directly with the body to shift your emotional state. By focusing on breathing exercises, movement, and touch, we can engage the PNS and restore a sense of safety. This allows the body to self-regulate and, through the mind-body connection, shift the emotional state of the mind.

It's only when you feel secure in your body that you can effectively engage the cognitive, rational part of your brain and engage in higher-level thinking, emotion regulation, and self-reflection to increase psychological resilience (which we will explore in the following sections of this chapter).

I am now going to introduce a few simple somatic exercises. These exercises are grouped into three categories.

1. **Calming:** Exercises to use when you notice you've shifted into a mobilized/sympathetic state to calm and bring you back to a relaxed state.

2. **Activating:** Exercises for when you're in an immobilized or dorsal vagal state and need activation to return to a regulated state.
3. **Daily practice:** Exercises to use regularly to tone the vagus nerve and help you stay in a relaxed state for longer.

I've provided several options. Try them all to see which ones work for you. I recommend spending a few minutes *daily* practicing the exercises from **daily practice**, and using the ones from **calming** and **activating** whenever your nervous system becomes dysregulated. With time and consistent practice, you will automatically start to respond to triggers with these techniques rather than reverting to the old, automatic patterns of dysregulation.

CALMING

Use these down-regulating techniques whenever you feel overly activated and are experiencing too much energy, tension, anxiety, or anger associated with the mobilized/sympathetic state (or hyperarousal). Try them all and stick with the ones that work best for you.

Diaphragmatic breathing

Multiple studies indicate that voluntary regulation of breathing can have a profound impact on psychological states and alleviate symptoms associated with anxiety, depression, and post-traumatic responses.[6] Deep, slow breathing accompanied by extended exhalation stimulates the vagus nerve, leading to a decrease in heart rate and blood pressure.

Diaphragmatic breathing is an easy practice for activating the vagus nerve and the PNS. By promoting slow, deep breaths, it helps to quickly down-regulate an overactive nervous system, overriding the sympathetic response, and bringing back a state of relaxation.

1. Sit or lie down.
2. Close your eyes or keep a soft gaze.
3. Put one hand on your belly and another on your chest.
4. Take a deep and slow breath through your nose. As you inhale, feel your belly expand. It should feel like it's gently pushing against the hand on your stomach.
5. Exhale slowly through your mouth, making your exhale longer than the inhale and allowing your belly to gently contract.
6. You can count the seconds of each to ensure the exhale is longer. For example, inhale for a count of 3–4 seconds and exhale for 5–6 seconds. Adjust the ratio to what feels comfortable for you.
7. Continue this deep belly breathing for 5–10 breaths.
8. After you finish, notice how you feel.

Cyclic sighing

Cyclic sighing—also known as the physiological sigh—is another simple breathing exercise that emphasizes long exhalations and can lower the heart rate and promote a sense of relaxation, mimicking the physiological benefits of a natural sigh. According to a study from Stanford Medicine, cyclic sighing might be more effective than other breathing methods for calming down.[7]

1. Sit down or stand up, whichever feels most comfortable for you.

2. Feel your lungs expand as you take a deep breath. Once you are nearly full, take a second, shorter inhale (a sharp, quick breath) to fully expand your lungs.
3. Exhale slowly through your mouth. Make it long and steady.
4. Repeat two or three times.
5. After you finish, take a moment to notice how you feel.

Five senses exercise

In this exercise, we'll use the body's sensory systems, specifically exteroception (see page 204), to ground and regulate in the present moment. This helps calm the nervous system by shifting your focus away from the noise in your mind and toward what's happening around you in reality. I find this exercise especially effective when the sensations in my body are overwhelming and are contributing to my dysregulation (such as a fast heart rate).

1. Sit down or stand up, whichever feels most comfortable for you.
2. Take a deep breath in through your nose and slowly exhale through your mouth. Start noticing your surroundings. We'll focus on each of your five senses.
3. Look around you and scan the room. Look at the windows, door, floor, and furniture, and notice the objects and details you haven't seen before, such as the texture of the curtains, the pattern on the rug, or the way the light falls on a surface.
4. Listen carefully to the sounds around you, both inside and outside the room.

5. Pay attention to what you can touch. Notice the feel of your clothes, the ground beneath your feet, or the chair you're sitting on.
6. What smells can you detect in the air? Take a moment to notice them.
7. Check in with the taste in your mouth. Is it from something you ate or drank, like toothpaste or coffee?
8. Take a deep breath in through your nose and out through your mouth to close the exercise and notice how you feel now.

Shaking

Involuntary shaking is a natural physiological response to intense stress, observed in both humans and animals. For example, after escaping a predator, animals often shake once they reach safety. This shaking is thought to help release the excess energy mobilized during the fight-or-flight response.

Voluntary shaking can mimic this natural process, supporting nervous system regulation by discharging pent-up energy and helping the body shift into a more balanced, relaxed state.

- Sit down comfortably on a chair with both feet flat on the ground.
- Focus on your hands first and give them a gentle shake for a few seconds.
- Gradually expand the movement to include your wrists and arms.

- Shift your attention to your legs, and gently start shaking both legs at the same time while keeping your feet on the ground.
- If you're comfortable, stand up and shake your whole body in any way that feels easy and natural to you, creating a rhythmic movement.
- After shaking, sit still for a moment and take note of how your body feels, noticing the contrast between the shaking and the calm.

ACTIVATING

Use these up-regulating techniques whenever you feel low energy, numb, sad, or dissociated in your immobilized/dorsal vagal state (or hypo-arousal). Try them all and stick with the ones that work best for you.

Tactile activation

By engaging in sensory stimulation through touch, this exercise promotes physical awareness, helping to "awaken" the sensory systems. This gradual activation of the nervous system can be particularly effective in breaking through numbness or dissociation, bringing you back into the moment and more energy to the body.

1. Stand up with your feet hip-width apart.
2. Rub your palms together to generate some heat.
3. Begin gently patting one arm with your hand. Start at your shoulder and work your way down to your elbow, fore-

arm, wrist, and hand. Then, come back up from underneath your arm to your armpit. Focus on the rhythm of the movement and the sensations in your body.

4. Switch to the other arm and repeat the same pattern.
5. Now, use both hands to gently tap your chest, then continue tapping down to your belly, around to your lower back, and finish at your buttocks.
6. Move to one of your legs, relax your body forward, and use both hands to pat your thigh. Keep rolling down your spine and continue patting your knee, shin and calf, and ankle as you fold forward.
7. Repeat the same process with the other leg.
8. Slowly roll back up to a straight position. Take a few seconds to notice the shift in energy through your body.

Mindful movement

Any type of gentle movement, such as walking, yoga, stretching, swaying, or dancing, engages proprioception (your sense of your body position and movement) and the vestibular sense (your sense of balance and spatial orientation). This helps reconnect you with your body and can be especially effective in alleviating feelings of immobilization and hypo-arousal.

1. Stand with your feet hip-width apart.
2. Slowly stretch your arms overhead as you inhale.
3. On the exhale, bring your arms down.
4. Repeat the motion of your arms going up and down 5–10 times, focusing on your breath and the sensations of moving your arms.

5. Stand straight with your arms down, and begin swaying gently from side to side, shifting your weight from one foot to the other. Move in a way that feels good to you and notice the rhythm and movement in your body. Continue for 1–2 minutes.
6. Next, slowly twist your torso from side to side, allowing your arms to follow the motion. Continue for another 1–2 minutes.
7. Pause, stand still and take a moment to check in with how your body feels now.

Music and movement

Upbeat music can influence brain activity, particularly in areas related to attention, arousal, and emotion regulation. When combined with movement, it can help bring more energy to the body and support a return to a more regulated state.

1. Choose an upbeat, fun song that you love.
2. Start dancing however feels good to you, letting the rhythm of the song guide your movements.
3. Keep moving with the music for the entire song, allowing your body to naturally follow the rhythm.
4. When the song finishes, pause and stand still for a moment. Check in with how your body feels now.

Breath of fire

You learned previously that breathing with long, slow exhales activates the PNS, helping to calm the body. The opposite is also true: Fast, shallow breathing with short exhales can activate the SNS, helping to bring energy when you're feeling sluggish or stuck in a low-energy state.

Breath of fire is an activating breathing technique commonly used in Kundalini yoga to move energy and awaken the body. Warning: Do not practice breath of fire if you are pregnant, have high blood pressure, or have any respiratory issues. Always stop if you feel dizzy or light-headed.

1. Sit down straight with your shoulders relaxed.
2. Close your eyes or keep a soft gaze.
3. Take a deep inhale into your belly through your nose.
4. Exhale forcefully through your nose while contracting your belly muscles as you exhale.
5. Focus on fast, forceful exhales by contracting your belly; your inhales will come naturally.
6. Continue for 30 seconds if you feel comfortable. Stop if you feel dizzy or light-headed.
7. Pause for a moment and check in with how your body feels now. Notice any shifts in energy.

DAILY PRACTICE

The following exercises are daily practices designed to tone your vagus nerve and support ventral vagal activity so you can stay in the relaxed state for longer periods. By incorporating them into your routine, you can expand your window of tolerance and increase your nervous system flexibility and resilience.

Experiment with each exercise and stick with those that bring the most benefits for you. Then, pick a specific time and place (cue) to practice consistently, making it part of your daily routine until it becomes a habit. For example, I like to do 12 Sun Salutations when I wake up in the morning. I have done them (almost) every single day for the last 10 years, and I don't even have to think about it! Let's see how this could work for you. Suppose resonance breathing resonates most with you, and you decide to practice it for 5–10 minutes daily. To make it stick, take advantage of the habit loop we explored in "How the Cortisol Reset Plan Will Help You Thrive":

Cue (on the train to work) → behavior (resonance breathing) → reward (calmer and more at peace)

Over time, as you repeat the habit, your brain recognizes the cue and initiates the response automatically, making it an effortless part of your routine.

Resonance breathing

Resonance breathing is breathing at a slow rate with the same inhale and exhale duration. The rate is usually 4.5–7 breaths per minute and it has been shown to increase HRV.[8] Remember, a higher HRV is associated with better ANS regulation (see page 35).

1. Sit down straight with your shoulders relaxed.
2. Close your eyes or keep a soft gaze.
3. Inhale through your nose for a count of 5 seconds.
4. Exhale slowly through your nose for a count of 5 seconds.
5. Continue for 5–10 minutes.
6. Ideally, practice once or twice daily.

Humming (Bhramari pranayama)

Humming engages the muscles of the throat, which are near the vagus nerve. This stimulation may promote vagal tone. Studies have shown that humming can lead to improved HRV.[9]

1. Sit down straight with your shoulders relaxed.
2. Close your eyes or keep a soft gaze.
3. Take a slow, deep inhale through your nose, expanding your chest and belly.
4. As you exhale, begin to hum, making a steady "mmmm" sound. Try to sustain the hum for the entire exhale, feeling the vibrations in your throat.
5. Continue humming for 5 minutes.

Half salamander exercise

This exercise, from Stanley Rosenberg's book *Accessing the Healing Power of the Vagus Nerve*, stimulates the vagus nerve and improves mobility in the neck and blood flow to the brain, which supports the ventral vagal branch of the vagus nerve that brings regulation.[10]

1. Sit down straight with your shoulders relaxed.
2. Without turning your head, look to the right.
3. Continue looking to the right side and tilt your head to the right, bringing your right ear toward your right shoulder (without lifting the shoulder).
4. Hold this position for 30 seconds.
5. Return to the neutral position with your neck and spine aligned and look forward.

6. Now, repeat on the other side. Look to the left and then tilt your head, bringing your left ear toward your left shoulder. Hold for another 30 seconds.
7. Return to an upright position and look forward.

Yoga Sun Salutations (Surya Namaskar)

Yoga can increase HRV and improve the balance between sympathetic and parasympathetic activity, contributing to better ANS regulation.[11] This quick and easy sequence can be done in fewer than 10 minutes, and it's a great start to the day.

If you're new to Sun Salutations, below are some steps to follow, but you may find it easier to use a video tutorial—there are plenty on YouTube.

1. Stand straight at the top of your yoga mat, with feet hip-width apart and arms at your sides (Mountain Pose).
2. Inhale and raise your arms overhead, bringing your palms together, reaching toward the sky.
3. Exhale and fold forward at the hips, bringing your hands to your shins, ankles or the floor (Forward Fold/Uttanasana).
4. Inhale and step back with one foot at a time into Plank pose. Your body should create a somewhat straight line (like a plank) from your head to your heels, with your shoulders stacked over your wrists.
5. Exhale as you lower yourself to the floor, either stopping halfway in Chaturanga with elbows bent at 90 degrees or lowering all the way to your belly while keeping your elbows close to your ribs.
6. Inhale and lift your chest into Cobra pose, keeping your elbows bent, or straighten them for Upward-Facing Dog.

7. Exhale and lift your hips and thighs up and back into Downward-Facing Dog.
8. Inhale and step your right foot forward between your hands.
9. Exhale and step your left foot forward to meet the right in Forward Fold.
10. Inhale and rise up, reaching your arms overhead and coming into a standing position.
11. Exhale and return to Mountain Pose with arms at your sides.
12. Repeat 12 rounds, alternating which foot steps forward first.

By cultivating awareness and tapping into your body's natural regulating systems, you learn to create a sense of safety within the body. This is very regulating and soothing by itself and helps reduce the activation of your stress response, supporting balanced cortisol levels.

Once you can self-regulate using your body, you can progress to the next two building blocks of psychological resilience and well-being—connecting to Self and others—by engaging the thinking part of the brain.

Connect to Self

In this building block, you will become a nonjudgmental and curious *observer* of the thoughts and narratives of your mind. As you become aware of the inner workings of the mind, you can start to identify, challenge, and modify limiting beliefs and maladaptive behaviors or coping mechanisms that are often linked to attachment wounds and unmet emotional needs.

To become an observer means to tap into a part of you that has the ability to notice and watch your thoughts, emotions, and behaviors without getting caught up by them. It can feel like watching a movie, where you are just a spectator who is able to experience what is happening without getting caught up in the drama. If you are an experienced meditator, you're likely familiar with this state of "awareness" or "consciousness" that is often referred to as the Self.

The concept of the "Self" is central to many psychotherapy, spiritual, and philosophical practices, and it's seen as the key to emotional resilience, healing, and spiritual growth. By becoming the observer, you "step back" from the noise of your mind and begin to experience inner peace. Michael A. Singer, in his book *The Untethered Soul,* puts it this way: "There is nothing more important to true growth than realizing that you are not the voice of the mind—you are the one who hears it."[12]

In the Internal Family Systems (IFS) model, developed by Dr. Richard Schwartz, the mind is considered to be made up of multiple protective and wounded subminds or "parts" that are led by a core Self.[13] The parts are constantly interacting inside you and they all have different thoughts, beliefs, emotions, and impulses. Underlying the parts is a core Self that has the qualities of curiosity, calm, confidence, compassion, creativity, clarity, courage, and connectedness (8 Cs) and patience, persistence, presence, perspective, and playfulness (5 Ps).

Parts in IFS are categorized into Exiles, Managers, and Firefighters:

- **Exiles** are wounded parts that carry painful emotions and memories, often stemming from developmental attachment wounds or unmet emotional needs. We try to repress or lock these parts away because they cause us too much pain.

- **Managers** are protective parts that try to control the environment to prevent Exiles from being triggered, aiming to avoid the pain (they do that with behaviors such as perfectionism, people-pleasing, or trying to control people around them).
- **Firefighters** are also protectors, but they step in when Exiles inevitably get triggered and cause pain, using coping mechanisms and sometimes extreme behaviors like substance abuse, overeating, or overworking to numb the emotional intensity.

Exiles carry *burdens* from past experiences, especially from *attachment wounds* or unmet emotional needs in childhood. These parts are also called the "inner child" and they are the ones that take in the extreme beliefs such as "I'm not good enough" or "I don't deserve love." This concept is similar to John Bowlby's *internal working models* in attachment theory, which are the mental frameworks we develop in childhood that shape how we see ourselves and others, and what to expect from relationships.[14]

At the heart of *attachment theory* is the idea that infants need a strong bond with at least one caregiver to survive and feel secure. A *secure attachment* forms when caregivers respond consistently to the child's needs, creating trust and safety. However, attachment wounds can occur when caregivers are inconsistent, unresponsive, neglectful, or emotionally unavailable, creating a sense of distrust and lack of safety. This might lead to the development of *insecure attachment* styles, such as anxious, avoidant, or disorganized, which influence how we relate to others in our relationships as adults. Understanding your attachment style can help you connect with others better, and we will discuss this further in the next section.

Healing attachment wounds involves deep work that goes beyond the scope of this book. However, by getting to know and building a compassionate relationship with all your parts and by connecting with your nonjudgmental and caring Self, you can cultivate the trust and safety that your nervous system needs. This sense of inner security supports nervous system regulation, reducing the constant activation of the stress response, balancing cortisol levels, and lowering allostatic load.

We will do this through two exercises. The first will help you get to know your "parts" without becoming identified with them. This will allow you to access your true Self, which can provide safety, love, compassion, and reassurance to these parts, liberating them from their protective roles.

In the early stages of healing, we focus on the protective parts (Managers and Firefighters) rather than the wounded Exiles or inner children. Protective parts, such as the inner critic or people-pleaser, have developed maladaptive coping mechanisms to avoid emotional pain. By working with these parts first, you can establish a sense of safety and trust without the overwhelm that can come up when working with Exiles directly. In the second exercise, we will assess and change maladaptive coping patterns that don't serve you anymore.

PARTS AND THE SELF EXERCISE

In this exercise, we will connect with the different "parts" of ourselves and embody the "Self." Remember, the Self is the compassionate, calm, and nonjudgmental observer that can hold space for all parts without becoming overwhelmed.

Step 1: Connect with your parts

- Sit down and close your eyes or keep a soft gaze.
- Focus on the protective parts that are showing up for you right now. These parts may come up as feelings, thoughts, beliefs, or impulses. For example, you might notice a part that acts as the "inner critic," telling you that you should be doing more or that you're not good enough. Or, you might observe a part that avoids confrontation at all costs, preventing you from speaking up when you need to. Or maybe you can observe a part that wants to please everyone and can't say no or a part filled with self-doubt that needs constant reassurance. You may also notice a part that feels anxious or scared about the future.
- Acknowledge each part with curiosity, noticing its feelings, thoughts, and beliefs. Don't try to change or judge them. Listen to them with compassion, and remember they are trying to keep you and all the other parts safe the best way they know how.

Step 2: Access the Self

- Now, imagine stepping back from these parts. Try to tap into the sense of awareness that is separate from the parts. This is your true Self, which is not defined by any one part.
- Imagine that the Self is a loving and calm presence sitting inside you, able to witness all the parts without becoming trapped in their stories or emotions.

- Connect with the qualities of the Self—curiosity, calm, confidence, compassion, courage, and patience—and notice how these qualities feel in your body. Embodying these qualities often brings a sense of spaciousness and safety.

Step 3: Create dialogue with your parts

- Now, engage in a dialogue with your parts. Ask them what they need from you in this moment. Do they feel neglected, tired, or angry? What would that part like you to know or understand?
- As you listen, offer reassurance and understanding to each part. Let them know they are not alone anymore and that you are listening. You might say to the anxious part, "I understand you are scared and worried, but I am here now and I can protect you," or to the perfectionist part, "I see you trying to control things, and I can offer you rest."

I recommend you practice this exercise regularly to deepen your connection with your parts. As your parts learn to trust you, they will feel safer in letting go of their protective roles by letting you, the Self, lead. This dialogue can be incredibly healing; it's like being a calm, caring parent who is attuned to a child's needs. As you support your parts, they can finally relax.

You can also use this exercise as you go through your day. For example, if you notice the inner critic's chatter, pause and connect with that part of you, just as a compassionate parent would check on their child. Listen to what it's trying to say, ask about its needs, and reassure it that you are there and it can rely on you.

ASSESS YOUR COPING MECHANISMS

Coping mechanisms are learned behaviors developed by your protective parts to make you feel better or numb emotional pain. For instance, having a glass of wine to relax after a tough day at the office or going for a run after work can both be considered coping mechanisms. These aren't inherently "good" or "bad" because they are both attempting to make you feel better. However, some coping mechanisms are potentially keeping you stuck in unhelpful patterns or leading to more dysregulation. By recognizing these behaviors with compassion instead of shame, you can understand their intent (to keep you safe) and start the process of shifting toward healthier, more supportive strategies.

The goal in this section is to equip you with a range of strategies that not only help you handle your triggers more effectively but also support your long-term nervous system health.

Step 1: Identify your coping mechanisms

Pause for a moment to reflect on the coping mechanisms you currently use and write them down in a notepad or the Notes app on your phone. Remember, there's no shame in recognizing coping strategies that may have long-term negative effects.

Step 2: Identify the cause and the intent

Ask yourself, "What emotion is this coping mechanism trying to protect me from?" or "What emotional need is this behavior attempting to meet?" For example, you might notice that you spend too much time on social media during weekends. You think about what could be causing this and realize that it helps you soothe feelings of loneliness after a recent breakup. You used to spend your weekends with your partner, and now, with more time alone and without the distraction of work, the weekends are tough.

Step 3: Explore alternatives

Let's shift our focus to expanding your coping mechanism toolkit. Once you've identified the cause (and the intent) behind each coping mechanism, brainstorm healthier alternatives that can meet the same need. For instance, in the example above, you could reach out to a friend for a walk or coffee, or consider starting a new hobby that connects you with people who share similar interests.

Below is a list of healthy coping mechanisms you can explore. It's always a good idea to try a few and see which ones work for you.

- Call a friend or family member who makes you feel good and safe.
- Go for a brisk walk in nature, a park, or a green space to connect with the outdoors.
- Start a new hobby or activity that involves some sort of physical movement like golf, tennis, or dancing.
- Start a new hobby that involves creativity like painting, drawing, or writing.
- Try grounding exercises, such as walking barefoot on grass or sand.
- Attend a yoga class or follow a yoga video at home.
- Do household chores such as cleaning your house or organizing your wardrobe.

- Take a hot bath.
- Find a new recipe and cook a delicious meal.
- Volunteer your time for a good cause.
- Take a nap.
- Use a mindfulness app or a guided meditation.
- Watch a comedy.
- Read a book.
- Brainstorm solutions to a problem and make a pros-and-cons list.

> **Remember:** For a habit to stick, it needs to give you a reward; it needs to make you feel better so you come back for more.

Step 4: Practice consistently

Incorporate these alternatives into your daily routine until they become automatic habits. For example, if you've noticed that you feel highly activated after work due to your demanding job and struggle to switch off, you can introduce a simple coping mechanism. Your cue could be leaving the office, and the new behavior could be going for a swim at the pool nearby or going for a brisk walk in a park. You may find that this helps you wind down almost instantly, leaving you feeling calmer and better able to transition into your evening with more ease (this is the reward). With consistency, this healthier coping mechanism can become a new, automatic habit that not only helps you feel better in the moment, but also provides emotional regulation in the long run.

Connect to Others

Connection to others is a sense of kinship and care that allows us to create positive interactions and build caring and meaningful relationships with others.[15]

Human beings are inherently social creatures. From an evolutionary perspective, our survival depended on our ability to interact with and help each other. Living in groups and supporting each other improved our chances of survival, and this is now hardwired into our biology.

Studies show that positive social connections are linked with longevity and decreased mortality.[16] People with strong social support systems are better equipped to cope with stress and adversity, less likely to experience depression, anxiety, and other mental health issues, and more likely to have better physical health. The Harvard Study of Adult Development, also known as the Grant Study, looked at what influences healthy ageing and well-being over a lifetime.[17] It showed how important social connections are for physical health and emotional well-being. The research shows that people with strong social connections tend to be happier, healthier, and more resilient.

In this section, we will explore ways to strengthen your ability to build social connections and foster a sense of kinship and belonging. We will start by identifying your attachment style, which will allow you to observe and challenge your "social construals" or the ways you perceive others. From there, we will focus on developing two qualities that will improve how you perceive others (appreciation and compassion) and two qualities that will help you build healthier and meaningful relationships (kindness and healthy boundaries).

As we saw earlier, according to attachment theory, early experiences and bonds with our caregivers shape how we view ourselves and others. From these early bonds, we develop certain patterns or *attachment styles* of relating to others in adulthood. Children with secure attachments are more likely to grow into adults who see others as reliable and themselves as worthy of love. In contrast, children with insecure attachments are more likely to view others as untrustworthy or unreliable and see themselves as less deserving of loving connections.

The four main attachment styles are:

1. **Secure:** People with a secure attachment style typically view others with trust; they know they can rely on others. They are comfortable giving and receiving and can build healthy and trusting relationships.
2. **Anxious:** People with an anxious attachment style often perceive relationships with anxiety, fearing abandonment or rejection. They tend to interpret others' actions as signs of rejection or abandonment, leading to a constant need for reassurance. They also tend to overcompensate to feel safe in relationships (people-pleasing or lack of boundaries are common in people with an anxious attachment style).
3. **Avoidant:** Those with an avoidant attachment style often view intimacy and emotional closeness as uncomfortable or intrusive. They tend to be very independent and fear relying on others.

4. **Disorganized:** This is a less common style, which is a combination of anxious and avoidant. People with a disorganized attachment style often simultaneously seek intimacy and push people away, struggle to trust others, and often see their relationships as unsafe.

IDENTIFY YOUR ATTACHMENT STYLE

Think about a recent disagreement or argument with someone close to you. This could be with a romantic partner, a family member, or a close friend. Now, take a moment to reflect on how you felt and how you acted during the argument.

Here is how each style might show up:

Secure:

- **Feelings:** You may have felt hurt, but you also felt confident in your ability to resolve the issue and maintain connection.

- **Behaviors:** You were open to communicating and willing to listen, and you were able to express your needs.

Anxious:

- **Feelings:** You likely felt hurt but also anxious and worried that the conflict would lead to abandonment or rejection. You might have felt you were not lovable and feared that the other person no longer cared for you.

- **Behaviors:** You might have sought reassurance or become overly clingy, apologizing or trying to please the other person.

Avoidant:

- **Feelings:** You might have felt frustrated and maybe even hurt but quickly withdrew or shut down emotionally.
- **Behaviors:** You likely distanced yourself either physically or emotionally, avoiding discussing the issue or ignoring it. You might have pretended that you were okay even though you weren't.

Disorganized:

- **Feelings:** You might have felt a confusing mix of hurt, fear of abandonment, and uncertainty, and felt unsure about the relationship's stability.
- **Behaviors:** You might have alternated between seeking closeness (wanting to talk things through) and pushing the other person away (shutting down or becoming defensive).

Understanding your attachment style can help you identify patterns in relationships and help you recognize how certain beliefs shape the lens through which you view others, which might not always reflect reality. By becoming aware of these patterns, you can challenge and change unhelpful perceptions, leading to better interactions and healthier relationships. This is crucial because relationship issues are some of the most common triggers of the stress response. When unresolved, they can keep our stress levels chronically elevated, disrupting cortisol balance and contributing to allostatic load. By improving the quality of our relationships, we reduce a major source of stress.

The next step is to strengthen certain qualities that will improve your perception of others—these are appreciation and empathy.

APPRECIATION

Appreciation is the ability to look for and recognize the good in others. Unfortunately, due to the brain's tendency toward negativity bias, we often focus more on negative than positive traits in others. For example, maybe you fixate on how your partner is messy in the kitchen or struggles to talk about their feelings, overlooking the many other ways they contribute to your relationship. This tendency to dwell on negative traits can lead to pain, disconnection, and isolation as we may start assuming the worst about others.

This tendency is further influenced by our attachment styles. For instance, someone with an anxious attachment style might be hyper-focused on small behaviors that seem to show a lack of interest, interpreting them as signs of rejection or abandonment.

To counteract this tendency, we can train ourselves to look for positive traits instead. This doesn't mean ignoring negative traits or behaviors; instead, it means looking at the big picture so we can see it all. When you do this, you often realize that the good greatly outweighs the bad!

Here is an exercise that will help you cultivate more appreciation:

- Pick someone in your life (your partner, a family member, a friend, or a colleague).
- Write down three positive traits you've noticed about this person. Be as specific as possible. For example, instead of

just saying "They're kind," you could say "They are kind because they brought me a home-cooked meal when I just had my baby."

- After listing these qualities, think about how these traits contribute to your relationship with this person and the positive impact they have on your life.
- Whenever you catch yourself focusing on a negative trait or behavior of this person, pause and remind yourself of the positive traits you've written down.
- If it feels right to you, you could tell them how much you appreciate having them in your life. Gratitude has been shown to lead to better levels of perceived social support and can strengthen the relationship by making the other person feel valued.[18]

COMPASSION

One mindset shift that can completely change the way you perceive others is realizing that everyone in this world, just like you, has their own struggles and they are trying their best to be happy and avoid suffering. Understanding this very human fact helps you view people's behaviors with more compassion and understanding.

This doesn't mean you have to condone or accept every behavior. Instead, it means you can put yourself in other people's shoes, understand where they are coming from, and recognize that they are doing the best they can at this moment, even if their best isn't what you would hope for. Just as we approach our internal "parts" with compassion, recognizing that even when their emotions and behaviors are disruptive, their purpose is to protect us and help us avoid pain, we can extend that same compassion to others.

Studies have shown that when we experience compassion, areas of the brain associated with positive emotions and social connection become activated.[19] By practicing compassion, both toward ourselves and others, we strengthen our relationships and enhance our own emotional resilience.

Let's now discuss how to improve the quality of your relationships: cultivating kindness and setting healthy boundaries.

KINDNESS

Kindness is one of the most powerful qualities in human interactions. At its core, it's about doing things for others without expecting anything in return.

Kindness helps build trust in relationships because it makes people feel valued and cared for. This often leads to reciprocity, because when we show kindness, others are more likely to do the same, creating more supportive relationships. Kindness shifts our mindset from "I'm on my own" to "We're in this together," which reduces feelings of isolation and strengthens our sense of belonging.

While the main goal of kindness is to benefit others, recent studies show that practicing kindness also brings many benefits to the person being kind! It has been linked to lower stress levels, increased resilience,[20] improved mental and physical health, stronger social bonds, and may even help slow biological ageing.[21]

Kindness is a skill that can be developed through practice. The more you do it, the more your capacity for it grows, just like building muscle. It is also contagious; research shows that even witnessing kindness indirectly can trigger people to be kinder themselves.[22] This inspires others to pay it forward and creates a ripple effect that can benefit the community as a whole.

There are several ways you can cultivate kindness in your daily life:

- Start by truly listening when others speak, showing them that you care and are fully present.
- Look for opportunities to help without being asked, like running an errand for a busy friend, helping a colleague with a project, bringing a home-cooked meal to someone who is sick, or offering to watch a friend's kids when they need a break.
- Support causes that resonate with you by donating to charities that align with your values.
- Sometimes even just taking a moment to reach out to a friend with a simple text, asking how they are and reminding them you are here for them, can make a big difference.

Another way to cultivate kindness is through loving-kindness meditation. This practice focuses on generating feelings of love, kindness, and compassion, starting with yourself and gradually extending to others: first to someone close to you, then to someone neutral, then to someone you may have difficulties with, and ultimately, to all human beings. While loving-kindness meditation has its origins in Buddhism, it has been popularized in modern times by mindfulness and meditation teachers, such as Sharon Salzberg.[23]

Here is an adaptation of lovingkindness meditation:

- Sit comfortably, close your eyes or keep a soft gaze, and take a few deep breaths.

- Begin with yourself. Place your hand over your heart and silently repeat the following phrases:

  "May I be happy."

  "May I be well."

  "May I be free of suffering."

- Next, bring to mind someone you are very close to, such as your partner, parents, or children. Repeat these phrases:

  "May you be happy."

  "May you be well."

  "May you be free of suffering."

- Now, think of someone neutral, someone you don't have strong positive or negative feelings toward. This could be an acquaintance or a person you see regularly, like the barista at the coffee shop. Send them the same lovingkindness:

  "May you be happy."

  "May you be well."

  "May you be free of suffering."

- Next, think of someone you may have challenging feelings toward. This can be someone you don't like very much or someone you have had issues with in the past. Offer them the same wishes:

  "May you be happy."

  "May you be well."

  "May you be free of suffering."

- Finally, extend lovingkindness to all humans everywhere and repeat:

  "May we all be happy."

  "May we all be well."

  "May we all be free of suffering."

- After you've sent lovingkindness to yourself and others, sit quietly for a few moments and notice how you feel.

HEALTHY BOUNDARIES

The second key to improving the quality of your relationships is setting healthy boundaries. It might seem like boundaries go against the previous quality, kindness, but in reality, the ability to set healthy boundaries is one of the kindest things you can do for yourself.

Boundaries are meant to protect your own needs and energy while also respecting other people's. When you set clear boundaries, you know what you're willing to accept and what you're not, making it easier to communicate without feeling guilty. Boundaries promote mutual respect, trust, and understanding, helping to prevent conflicts and resentment in your relationships.

For some, especially those with an anxious attachment style, setting boundaries can feel tough. You might have an underlying belief that, in order to be loved and accepted, you need to please everyone. But overcommitting and saying yes to everything often leads to exhaustion and resentment, eventually hurting both you and your relationships. In my work with clients, I've consistently observed a strong link between a lack of clear boundaries and chronic stress, cortisol dysregulation, and burnout.

An effective strategy for setting boundaries is to tune in to your feelings when someone asks you to do something. If your immediate reaction is a strong inner voice saying, "No, I don't want to do that," then it's important to honor that instinct and say no outright when asked. Here are some ways you can say no with kindness:

- "Thank you for thinking of me, but I can't do that right now."
- "I wish I could help, but unfortunately I have other commitments."
- "I'm not the best fit for that task, but I can help you find someone else who is."

Another helpful strategy is to write down your boundaries. This can make it easier to say no and communicate your limits clearly to others:

1. **Reflect on your limits:** Take some time to reflect on what makes you feel uncomfortable and identify areas in which you may need to set boundaries. For example, think about how you feel when a colleague expects you to respond to work emails on the weekend. You can also think about past experiences where your boundaries were crossed, but maybe you didn't communicate them clearly and that led to resentment.
2. **Define your boundaries:** Based on your reflections, write down a few clear boundaries you want to establish. Be specific about what is unacceptable to you, and consider how you want to communicate these boundaries. For example, you could decide that it's not okay for your colleague to expect you to reply to emails on the weekends and that this is a boundary you want to create.
3. **Communicate your boundaries:** Now, start communicating what your boundaries are. Try to be kind but firm, and don't be afraid to restate your boundaries when they are crossed. Try not to make it about them but about you when you express your boundaries. For example, you could say: "When I check my work emails on the weekend, I feel drained. I won't be looking at my inbox so I can switch off and rest, but I will get back to you as soon as possible on Monday morning."

The beauty of setting boundaries is that, most of the time, you only need to set them once. People tend to respect them once they've been clearly communicated and understood.

And lastly, an important part of setting healthy boundaries is being mindful of the people you spend time with. If spending time with someone leaves you feeling drained or if you can't truly be yourself with them, try to limit the time you spend together. You don't need to be friends with everyone, and not everyone needs to like you! Instead, focus on those who make you feel good and invest more in nurturing those relationships.

Before we move on to the fifth building block of psychological resilience, let's think about how you can connect to Self and others this week. For example, if you notice your inner critic chattering in your mind, can you bring awareness to that part of you? Rather than identifying with it, can you listen to it with curiosity and compassion, and bring your Self into the conversation? Remember, the Self is a loving and calm presence within you. Equally, think about how you can bring more *appreciation* and *compassion* into your interactions with others. If someone's behavior upsets you, can you pause and see the bigger picture? Is it truly an issue or can you focus on their positive traits? Can you step into their shoes to understand them better? Can you think of simple ways to practice *kindness*—maybe a quick text to check on a friend is just what they need. And what about healthy *boundaries*? Could saying no to a project that doesn't align with your goals help you honor your needs?

Spend Time in Nature

The fifth building block of psychological resilience is connection to nature. Humans have an innate desire to spend time in nature, rooted in the fact that we have spent most of our evolutionary history closely connected to it. We have relied on nature for survival, providing food, water, energy, medicine, and more. Beyond survival, nature has also been a constant source of wonder and inspiration, influencing art and culture for millennia.

However, with the rise of urbanization, many people now spend less time in nature, leading to a growing disconnection from the natural world. This disconnection has been linked to negative effects on both physical and mental health, as well as reduced awareness of environmental issues, which may in turn change their level of commitment to protect the natural environment.

A recent review of 832 studies showed that physical and psychological connection to nature can have many benefits for our mental and physical well-being, including reducing stress, improving mood, boosting immune function, enhancing cognitive function, and improving our attitudes toward environmental conservation.[24]

Our physical connection to nature involves actively engaging with natural environments. This could include things like walking in a park, swimming in the ocean or a lake, hiking in the woods, or camping in the wild. On the other hand, our psychological connection to nature is about the emotional and spiritual bond we have with the natural world. It's about feeling awe and wonder. For example, when you watch a breathtaking sunset or look up at the stars at night, you may experience a sense of being part of something bigger than yourself.

By nurturing your connection to nature and embracing the feeling of awe it inspires, you can feel belonging and interconnectedness with the world around you, which will support emotional resilience.

Here are a few practices to deepen your connection to nature:

- **Spend more time outdoors:** Make sure you spend some time outdoors each day, whether it's going for a walk in a local park, going to the beach, sitting in a garden, or simply taking a few moments to look up at the sky and the clouds.
- **Use your exteroception skills:** Pay attention to your senses and notice the sights, sounds, smells, and sensations of nature. Listen to the wind, the chirping of birds or the sound of waves at the beach. Take in the colors around you like the green leaves of the tree, the blue water of the river, or the colorful flowers in the garden. Inhale deeply and enjoy the scents of nature, and run your fingers over the grass, the water, or the sand.
- **Plan more outdoor activities:** Try new outdoor activities that allow you to interact with nature, such as hiking, camping, or gardening.

What's the simplest way for you to connect with nature this week? Maybe you can spend some time in a park—looking at the trees, listening to the birds, and feeling the wind on your face. Or, if you're lucky enough to live near a river or ocean, you could take a few minutes to watch the water and the horizon, listening to the sound of the waves or tide.

Find Your Purpose

The last building block of emotional resilience is purpose. Purpose is what gives your life meaning and direction, and you can cultivate it by understanding better what really matters to you (your values) and then aligning your actions, decisions, and daily behaviors with those core values.

When you're connected to your purpose, you can see the bigger picture, make better decisions, and stay aligned with who you are, which will give you the confidence you need to keep going, even when things get tough.

Having a sense of purpose has many health benefits, too. Studies show that people with a strong sense of purpose tend to live longer,[25] experience fewer chronic health issues, and show lower levels of stress, better mental health, and resilience.[26]

To find your purpose, start by asking yourself these questions:

- **When do I feel most fulfilled?** Identify the things that make you feel joy and fulfillment. This could be time with loved ones, being in nature, or doing a specific type of work.
- **What truly matters to me in life?** This could include helping others, achieving career milestones, or having a positive impact on the environment or society.
- **What are my values?** Reflect on the values that are most important to you. These could be integrity, authenticity, kindness, community, compassion, courage, personal growth, creativity, justice, or learning.

Now, think about goals that align with those values. For example, if community is one of your values, you could set a goal to regularly volunteer in your community. Keep checking if your daily actions are in alignment with these values. Make changes when necessary to ensure your actions align with your values and, when faced with challenging decisions, ask yourself: "If I say yes, will this bring me closer to the life I really want?"

Living in alignment with your values builds a sense of safety, stability, and trust in yourself, which is very healing for the nervous system. Not only will you decrease stress, but you'll also build greater resilience to whatever comes your way, reducing the chronic activation of the stress response and helping keep cortisol levels in check. On the other hand, constantly making choices that go against your values can lead to internal conflict, emotional distress, and more stress.

• • •

Before we finish this chapter, I want to acknowledge that this final step—building emotional resilience—is likely the most involved in the entire five-step plan. I encourage you to look at this work as a continuous journey of personal growth and development rather than a quick fix.

Key Habits to Incorporate in Step Five

It would be unrealistic to expect yourself to achieve complete emotional resilience after just 2 weeks of implementing the habits in this chapter. However, below I have included a checklist with some prompts to get you started. Please revisit this step again and again to refine your skills.

Week 9

Hopefully, by now, the habits from the previous steps have become engrained and you're really noticing a difference in your energy levels and have boosted your "stress bucket" capacity. This week, let's focus on the first two pillars of psychological resilience—awareness and connection to your body. Remember to harness the power of the habit loop we discussed in "How the Cortisol Reset Plan Will Help You Thrive" (page 53) to integrate new practices into your day.

- ☐ Awareness: Take a few moments throughout each day to notice your body sensations, thoughts, and emotions. Pay attention to your breathing, whether you are clenching your jaw, the tension in your shoulders, and your posture. Notice the sensations in your belly, chest, and throat. Now, listen to your thoughts from your observing Self (remember, you are not your thoughts; you are the one listening to them): Are they negative, positive, or neutral? Can you identify any emotion? What is your nervous system state? Relaxed, mobilized, or immobilized?
- ☐ Connection to your body: If you identify your nervous system as either mobilized or immobilized, use one of the body practices to help you return to a regulated state (choose a relaxing practice when mobilized or an activating one when immobilized).
- ☐ Daily somatic practice: Incorporate one of the activities in the daily practice section (see pages 228–32). Choose the same time every day, like after waking up or after work.

Week 10

This week, let's build on the work you've done and start to address the remaining four pillars of psychological resilience—connection to Self, connection to others, time in nature, and finding your purpose. Don't forget to keep practicing the daily body regulation exercises from last week.

- ☐ Connection to Self: Take a moment this week to identify the "parts" that are most active. What do they need? Embody the qualities of the Self : curiosity, calm, confidence, compassion, creativity, clarity, courage, and connectedness (8 Cs), and patience, persistence, presence, perspective, and playfulness (5 Ps), and let your "parts" know that you are here like a caring parent who can provide support. If further regulation is needed, choose a healthy coping mechanism from the list provided on page 239.

- ☐ Connection to others: Try to practice appreciation, compassion, kindness, and healthy boundaries daily. For example, listen and pay attention when someone talks to you, do something kind without being asked, express gratitude, practice a loving-kindness meditation, remember the positive traits of someone when they do something that annoys you, or say no to protect your boundaries.
- ☐ Time in nature: Spend a few minutes in nature each day. You could incorporate this into your daily walk from Step Four and take a walk in a park during lunch, or you might prefer a weekend hike or beach visit.
- ☐ Finding your purpose: Revisit the questions on page 256 and start thinking about how you can live in alignment with your values. Reflect at the end of each day on whether your actions aligned with your purpose. If not, consider what you could do differently the next day.

For some people, seeking additional professional support from a therapist can be very beneficial. I want to acknowledge the importance of honoring that path, knowing that the skills you've learned in this step can complement and potentially accelerate your healing process.

Now that we've completed the five steps of the plan, take a moment to revisit the questionnaires on pages 47–50 and reflect on your symptoms. Compare your results from this week with those from week 1. Is your total score lower than it was at the beginning? A downward shift suggests that your symptoms are becoming less frequent or intense—which is exactly what we're aiming for. Are you feeling more energetic? Sleeping better? Experiencing fewer cravings, less bloating, or a calmer mind? Some improvements may be obvious, while others are more subtle or gradual—but all are signs that you're moving in the right direction.

This marks the end of the plan, but it's also the beginning of a lifestyle—and in Part III I've included some delicious recipes that will not only nourish your body but will support your transformation in the months ahead.

Part III

The Cortisol Reset Recipes

Welcome to Part III of the Cortisol Reset Plan. Some of you have completed all five steps, while others are coming straight from Step One or Two, using this section to put into practice what you've learned as you continue working through the remaining steps in Part II. If you've completed all five steps and used the recipes as needed, feel free to skip ahead to the final section of the book, "Moving Forward" (page 298). And if you're still working through the plan, this section is here to support you in applying what you've learned so far and turning it into real-life meals. I encourage you to use these recipes as a starting point to build confidence in establishing a solid foundation for your eating habits. As you become more familiar with this way of eating, you'll be creating a long-term framework that will serve you well for years to come. These meals are here to guide you initially, but the ultimate goal is to empower you to make healthy meal choices that work for you beyond this plan.

Each recipe includes nutrient-dense ingredients to nourish your body and also a good balance of protein, fiber-rich carbohydrates, and fats to support balanced blood sugar levels. Whether you follow the recipes closely or use them as inspiration for your own creations, the choice is yours!

Note: The calorie and macro values are estimates and may vary depending on the brand or type of ingredients you use. Unless otherwise specified, there is no need to peel the vegetables or fruits if they're organic (you'll obtain more fiber that way!).

Breakfast

Blueberry and Cottage Cheese Oatmeal

Serves 1

Ingredients

¼ cup dry rolled oats

⅔ cup cottage cheese

1 tablespoon protein powder

¼ cup blueberries

Method

1. Cook the oats according to the instruction on the package, adding enough water so they stay creamy and don't get too thick.
2. Mix the cottage cheese and protein powder together in a bowl. Add the cooked oats and stir well. If it's too thick, add a splash of water or milk to reach your desired consistency.
3. Top with the blueberries and enjoy!

PROTEIN ~30 GRAMS, CARBS ~29 GRAMS, FAT ~8 GRAMS

Salmon and Sweet Potato Breakfast Hash

Serves 1

Ingredients

1 teaspoon avocado oil or extra-virgin olive oil

1 medium sweet potato, diced into ½-inch pieces

½ celery stalk, finely chopped

½ yellow onion, finely chopped

¼ pound skinless wild salmon fillet, coarsely chopped

1 tablespoon fresh dill, chopped (plus extra to garnish)

1 teaspoon fresh thyme leaves

Sea salt and black pepper, to taste

Method

1. Heat the oil in a skillet over medium heat. Add the sweet potato, celery, and onion to the pan. Sauté for about a minute.
2. Cover the skillet and cook for 5–7 minutes. Stir halfway through to ensure even cooking.
3. Remove the lid and increase the heat to medium-high. Add the salmon, dill, thyme leaves, sea salt, and black pepper to the skillet.
4. Stir the mixture frequently for 5–8 minutes, allowing the potatoes to lightly brown and the salmon to cook through.
5. Once the salmon is cooked and the potatoes are tender, remove the skillet from the heat.
6. Garnish with additional chopped fresh dill if desired.

PROTEIN 29 GRAMS, CARBS 34 GRAMS, FAT 17 GRAMS

Pre- and Probiotic Smoothie

Serves 1

Ingredients

½ cup unsweetened plain kefir

1 small banana

⅓ cup frozen mixed berries

1 tablespoon ground flaxseeds

1 teaspoon chia seeds

3 tablespoons protein powder

Pinch of ground cinnamon

Method

1. Add the kefir, banana, frozen berries, flaxseeds, chia seeds, protein powder, and cinnamon to a blender with ¼ cup of water.
2. Blend until smooth.
3. Taste and add another ¼ cup of water if necessary, depending on the consistency you like.
4. Pour into a glass.

PROTEIN 32 GRAMS, CARBS 44 GRAMS, FAT 8.5 GRAMS

Egg and Black Bean Breakfast Taco

Serves 1

Ingredients

3 large eggs

1 teaspoon avocado or extra-virgin olive oil

⅓ cup black beans (cooked or tinned), drained and rinsed

Sea salt, to taste

2 small corn (or whole-wheat) tortillas

⅓ cup cherry tomatoes, cut in half or quarters

¼ cup chopped fresh cilantro leaves, to garnish

Avocado (optional)

Method

1. In a small bowl, whisk the eggs.
2. Heat a skillet over medium-low heat. Once the skillet is hot, add the oil and pour in the whisked eggs. Stir continuously until the eggs are almost fully cooked.
3. Stir in the black beans and cook for another 30 seconds to finish cooking the eggs and heat the beans through.
4. Add a pinch of salt.
5. Assemble the tacos by placing the egg and black bean mixture onto the tortillas.
6. Add the chopped tomatoes and cilantro on top and serve.

Optional: Spread a little mashed avocado on the tortillas before adding the filling.

PROTEIN 28 GRAMS, CARBS 40 GRAMS, FAT 21 GRAMS

Overnight Quinoa and Raspberry Yogurt Bowl

Serves 1

Ingredients

1 cup plain Greek yogurt

¼ cup milk (dairy or alternative)

¼ cup quinoa flakes

1 tablespoon hemp seeds

½ teaspoon ground cinnamon

1 teaspoon honey

⅓ cup raspberries

1 tablespoon pumpkin seeds

Method

1. In a bowl, combine the yogurt, milk, quinoa flakes, hemp seeds, cinnamon, and honey.
2. Mix well until all ingredients are evenly combined and put it in the fridge overnight.
3. Top the yogurt mixture with the raspberries and pumpkin seeds, and enjoy!

PROTEIN 31 GRAMS, CARBS 39 GRAMS, FAT 14 GRAMS

Scrambled Eggs, Chicken Sausage, and Sautéed Veggies

Serves 1

Ingredients

1 teaspoon extra-virgin olive or avocado oil

3 ounces organic chicken sausage

1 cup white button mushrooms, sliced

2 cups fresh baby spinach

Sea salt and black pepper, to taste

2 large eggs

1 orange, peeled and cut into segments, to serve

Method

1. Heat the oil in a medium-sized skillet over medium heat.
2. Add the chicken sausage and cook for 8–10 minutes until browned and fully cooked through, turning occasionally. Remove from the skillet and set aside.
3. In the same pan, add the sliced mushrooms and sauté for about 3 minutes, until softened.
4. Add the fresh spinach and cook for another 1 minute, until wilted.
5. Season with a pinch of sea salt and black pepper. Remove from the skillet and set aside with the sausage.
6. In a bowl, whisk the eggs.
7. Pour the eggs into the same skillet over medium-low heat, stirring occasionally until they are just set and fluffy. Add a pinch of sea salt and black pepper.
8. On a plate, layer the scrambled eggs, sausage, sautéed mushrooms, and spinach.
9. Serve with the fresh orange segments on the side.

PROTEIN 31 GRAMS, CARBS 20 GRAMS, FAT 27 GRAMS

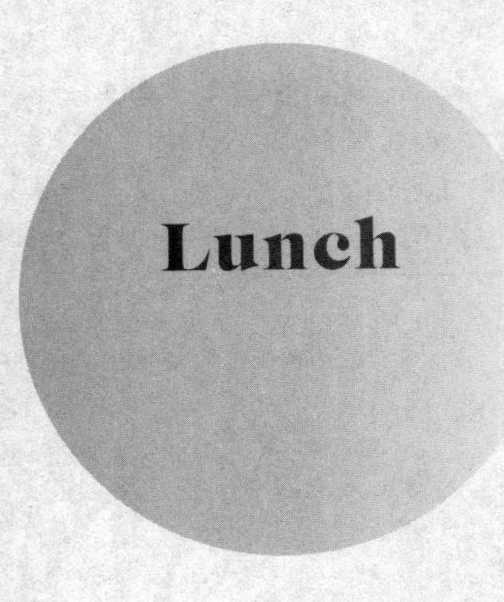

Lunch

Hearty Chicken, Vegetable, and White Bean Soup

Serves 4

Ingredients

1 tablespoon avocado oil

1 large yellow onion, chopped

1 large celery stalk, chopped

2 medium carrots, peeled and diced

1 medium zucchini, chopped

1 cup pumpkin, peeled and diced

4 garlic cloves, minced

2 teaspoons dried oregano

1 pound skinless chicken breast or thigh fillets, chopped into small pieces

6 cups Chicken Bone Broth (page 295)

3 cups finely chopped kale

2 cups white beans, cooked or from a can

Sea salt and black pepper, to taste

Juice of ½ lemon

Method

1. Heat the oil in a large pot over medium-high heat. Add the onion and cook for 3–5 minutes until softened.
2. Add the celery, carrots, zucchini, pumpkin, garlic, and oregano, and cook for another 3–5 minutes, stirring often.
3. Add the chicken and bone broth, bringing the mixture to a boil.
4. Once boiling, reduce the heat to low and simmer for about 20–30 minutes, until the pumpkin is soft.
5. Add the finely chopped kale and cook for another 5 minutes.
6. Stir in the white beans and cook 1 more minute until warmed through.

7. Season with salt and pepper to taste
8. Squeeze the lemon juice into the soup and season with additional salt and pepper if needed.
9. Ladle the soup into bowls and serve hot.

PROTEIN 39 GRAMS, CARBS 30 GRAMS, FAT 11 GRAMS

Shrimp and Quinoa Bowl

Serves 2

Ingredients

½ pound shrimp, peeled and deveined

1 teaspoon sweet paprika

1 teaspoon avocado oil

Sea salt and black pepper, to taste

1 cup cooked quinoa

½ red bell pepper, diced

1 medium cucumber, diced

1 cup arugula

2 spring onions, thinly sliced

1 tablespoon extra-virgin olive oil

Juice of 1 lemon

Method

1. In a mixing bowl, combine the shrimp with the sweet paprika and avocado oil. Season with salt and pepper to taste.
2. Heat a skillet or a pan over medium heat. Add the seasoned shrimp to the skillet and cook for 2–3 minutes per side, until cooked through.
3. Divide the cooked quinoa between two serving bowls.
4. Top the quinoa with the cooked shrimp, red bell pepper, cucumber, arugula, and spring onions.
5. Drizzle olive oil and lemon juice over the bowls.
6. Adjust the seasoning with additional salt and pepper if needed.

PROTEIN 34 GRAMS, CARBS 30 GRAMS, FAT 13 GRAMS

Tempeh and Avocado Salad with Tahini Dressing

Serves 2

Ingredients

8 ounces tempeh, sliced into strips or cubes

2 teaspoons extra-virgin olive oil, divided

Sea salt and black pepper, to taste

2 cups mixed leafy greens

6 radishes, thinly sliced

½ cup sugar snap peas, sliced

1 carrot, grated

1 tablespoon tahini

1 teaspoon lemon juice

1 teaspoon tamari

½ ripe avocado, peeled, destoned and sliced

2 tablespoons hemp seeds

Method

1. Cook the tempeh in a pan with 1 teaspoon oil for 5–7 minutes, stirring occasionally, until golden and crispy. Season with salt and pepper.
2. In a large bowl, combine the mixed leafy greens and the radishes, sugar snap peas, and carrot.
3. In a small bowl, whisk together the tahini, lemon juice, tamari, 1 teaspoon olive oil, and a pinch of salt and pepper. Add water to adjust the dressing's consistency to your liking.
4. Once the tempeh is done, remove it from the pan and let it cool slightly. Add the tempeh to the salad bowl.
5. Drizzle the tahini dressing over the salad and toss gently to coat everything.
6. Top with sliced avocado and hemp seeds.

PROTEIN 29 GRAMS, CARBS 26 GRAMS, FAT 26 GRAMS

Lentil Soup with Turkey Meatballs

Serves 4

Ingredients

1 pound ground turkey

2 garlic cloves, minced

Sea salt and black pepper, to taste

2 teaspoons avocado oil

1 yellow onion, sliced

1 fennel bulb, sliced

2 medium leeks, thinly sliced

5 cups Chicken Bone Broth (page 295)

2 cups cooked brown or green lentils, or about 2 cans, drained and rinsed

1 cup chopped fresh parsley

Method

1. Prepare the turkey meatballs first. In a bowl, mix the ground turkey with the garlic and some salt and pepper. Roll the mixture into small meatballs. Set aside.
2. Heat the oil in a pot over medium-high heat. Add the onion, fennel, and leeks. Sauté for about 10 minutes, or until they become soft and translucent.
3. Pour in the bone broth and season with salt and pepper. Stir well and bring the soup to a simmer.
4. Add the turkey meatballs to the simmering soup. Cover the pot with a lid and let it simmer for about 15 minutes.
5. Remove the lid and add the lentils to the pot. Stir gently and let the soup simmer uncovered for another 10 minutes.
6. Once the soup is ready, remove it from the heat and stir in the parsley.
7. Divide the soup among serving bowls and enjoy!

PROTEIN 40 GRAMS, CARBS 36 GRAMS, FAT 15 GRAMS

Chicken Salad Wrap

Serves 1

Ingredients

3.5 ounces rotisserie chicken, shredded

1 celery stick, finely chopped

¼ small red onion, finely chopped

2 tablespoons finely chopped fresh parsley

3 tablespoons plain Greek yogurt

Juice and zest of ½ lemon

1 teaspoon Dijon mustard

Sea salt and black pepper, to taste

½ cup arugula

1 brown rice tortilla

Method

1. In a medium-sized bowl, combine the chicken, celery, red onion, parsley, yogurt, lemon juice, lemon zest, Dijon mustard, sea salt, and black pepper. Mix well until all the ingredients are evenly incorporated.
2. Place the arugula on the tortilla.
3. Spoon the chicken salad mixture onto the tortilla over the arugula.
4. Roll up the tortilla tightly to form a wrap.
5. Slice the wrap in half, if desired, and serve immediately.

PROTEIN 37 GRAMS, CARBS 34 GRAMS, FAT 10 GRAMS

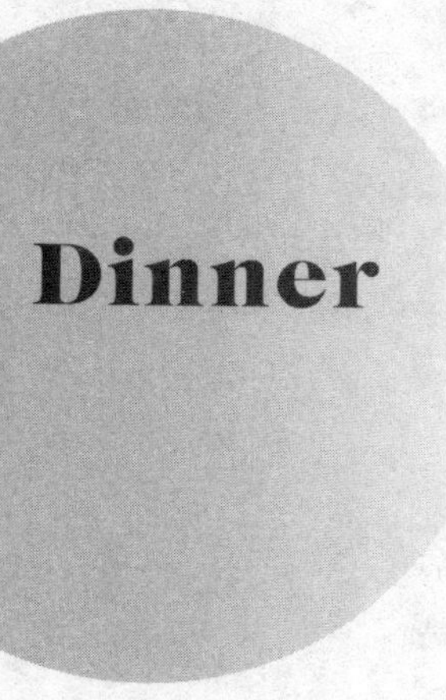

Dinner

Poached Salmon, Artichokes, and Sweet Potato

Serves 2

Ingredients

2 cups Chicken Bone Broth (page 295)

1 sweet potato, diced

2 garlic cloves, chopped

⅔ pound skinless salmon fillet

1 cup marinated artichoke hearts, drained and halved

3 spring onions, sliced

Juice of ½ lemon

½ cup chopped fresh parsley or dill

Sea salt and black pepper, to taste

Method

1. In a shallow pan, bring the broth to a boil. Add the sweet potato and garlic. Cover and simmer for 5 minutes.
2. Carefully add the salmon fillet, artichoke hearts, and spring onions to the pan. Cover and continue cooking for an additional 4–7 minutes, or until the salmon is fully cooked and the sweet potato is tender.
3. Once cooked, remove from heat and stir in the lemon juice. Add fresh herbs on top and season with sea salt and black pepper to taste.
4. Divide into bowls and serve immediately.

PROTEIN 38 GRAMS, CARBS 26 GRAMS, FAT 20 GRAMS

Roasted Herb Chicken and Veggies

Serves 4

Ingredients

3 medium potatoes, diced

1 zucchini, sliced

1 red bell pepper, sliced

2 small or 1 big broccoli head, cut into florets

1 red onion, sliced

2 teaspoons extra-virgin olive oil, divided

1 teaspoon dried oregano

½ teaspoon dried thyme

½ teaspoon smoked paprika

Sea salt and black pepper, to taste

1 pound skinless chicken breast or thigh fillets, cut into chunks

Juice of ½ lemon

½ cup chopped fresh parsley or basil, to garnish

Method

1. Preheat the oven to 400°F and line a baking tray with parchment paper.
2. In a large bowl, toss the potato, zucchini, red bell pepper, broccoli, and onion with 1 teaspoon of oil, oregano, thyme, paprika, and some salt and pepper.
3. In a separate bowl, coat the chicken pieces with the remaining oil and some salt and pepper.
4. Spread the veggies onto the lined tray.
5. Add the chicken pieces on top of the veggies.
6. Roast for 25–30 minutes, until the chicken is cooked through and the potatoes are golden and tender.
7. Squeeze lemon juice over the tray and garnish with fresh parsley or basil.
8. Serve warm and enjoy!

PROTEIN 39 GRAMS, CARBS 38 GRAMS, FAT 10 GRAMS

Honey Garlic Pork Meatballs with Asparagus and Carrots

Serves 4

Ingredients

1 pound lean ground pork

4 garlic cloves, minced and divided

1 tablespoon grated fresh root ginger

4 spring onions, sliced and divided

1 teaspoon sea salt

1 bunch (about 20 spears) asparagus, chopped into bite-sized pieces

2 medium carrots, diced

2 tablespoons tamari

1 tablespoon apple cider vinegar

2 tablespoons honey

1 teaspoon arrowroot powder

Method

1. Preheat the oven to 375°F. Line a baking tray with parchment paper.
2. In a large bowl, mix together the pork, half of the garlic, the ginger, two-thirds of the spring onions, and sea salt. Use your hands to combine the ingredients well. Shape the mixture into golf ball–size meatballs and place them on the lined tray. Bake in the oven for 18–20 minutes, flipping halfway through, until cooked through.
3. While the meatballs are baking, steam the asparagus and carrots together over boiling water for about 5 minutes, until just tender.
4. In a medium-sized pot, combine the remaining garlic, tamari, apple cider vinegar, and honey. In a small bowl, mix the arrowroot powder and 2 tablespoons of water until smooth, then add it to the pot. Bring the mixture to a low boil over medium heat, then reduce the heat and simmer for 2–3 minutes, until the sauce thickens.

5. Once the meatballs are cooked, toss them in the sauce until evenly coated. Divide the meatballs onto plates with the steamed asparagus and carrots. Sprinkle with the remaining sliced spring onions.

PROTEIN 28 GRAMS, CARBS 25 GRAMS, FAT 19 GRAMS

Baked White Fish with Zucchini and Baby Potatoes

Serves 2

Ingredients

6–8 baby potatoes, halved

1 tablespoon avocado oil

Salt and pepper, to taste

2 fillets (approximately 5 ounces each) sole, haddock, cod, flounder, or another mild white fish

2 medium zucchinis, sliced

2 tablespoons capers, drained and rinsed

1 tablespoon chopped fresh dill, to garnish

Juice of ½ lemon

Method

1. Preheat the oven to 425°F. Place the baby potatoes in a baking dish. Drizzle with the oil, toss to coat evenly, and season with salt and pepper.
2. Bake in the oven for 20 minutes, until the potatoes are slightly golden and tender.
3. Remove the baking dish from the oven and add the fish fillets and zucchini. Sprinkle the capers over the top.
4. Lower the oven temperature to 400°F and return the baking dish to the oven. Bake for another 15–20 minutes, or until the fish is cooked through and flakes easily with a fork.
5. Garnish with fresh dill and a squeeze of lemon juice before serving.

PROTEIN 34 GRAMS, CARBS 30 GRAMS, FAT 10 GRAMS

Hearty Beef, Mushroom, and Pea Stew

Serves 4

Ingredients

1 tablespoon extra-virgin olive oil

1 pound lean stewing beef (or lean chuck)

1 onion, diced

2 garlic cloves, minced

2 carrots, sliced

2 celery stalks, sliced

2 cups mushrooms, sliced

1 tablespoon tomato puree

1 tablespoon finely chopped fresh rosemary (or 1 teaspoon dried rosemary)

1 teaspoon sea salt

½ teaspoon black pepper

5 cups Beef Bone Broth (page 294)

2 cups peas (fresh or frozen)

1 tablespoon apple cider vinegar

½ cup chopped fresh parsley, to garnish

Method

1. Heat the oil in a large pot over medium heat. Add the beef and brown on all sides, about 5 minutes. Remove the beef and set aside.
2. In the same pot, add the onion, garlic, carrots, and celery, sautéing for about 5 minutes, until softened.
3. Add the mushrooms, cooking for another 5 minutes.
4. Stir in the tomato puree, rosemary, salt, and pepper. Cook for 2 minutes.
5. Add the browned beef back into the pot with the bone broth. Bring to a boil, then reduce to a simmer. Cover and let cook for 30 minutes, or until the beef is tender.

6. Add the peas and cook for an additional 5–10 minutes.
7. Stir in the apple cider vinegar and adjust the seasoning to taste.
8. Serve the stew in bowls, garnished with fresh parsley.

PROTEIN 37 GRAMS, CARBS 21 GRAMS, FAT 19 GRAMS

High-Protein Mini Chickpea Pizzas

Serves 2 (3 mini pizzas each)

Ingredients

1 can (15 oz) cooked chickpeas, drained and rinsed

2 large eggs

Pinch of salt

2–3 tablespoons tomato passata (or tomato sauce of your choice)

½ cup mozzarella cheese (shredded)

Toppings (choose your favorites):

3 ounces rotisserie chicken (shredded)

1 ½ cups fresh veggies (e.g., bell peppers, mushrooms, onions), sliced

1 teaspoon dried oregano

Basil leaves

Method

1. Preheat the oven to 350°F. Line a baking tray with parchment paper.
2. Dry the chickpeas with a towel to remove excess moisture.
3. In a food processor, blend the eggs, chickpeas, and a pinch of salt until smooth.
4. Spoon the mixture onto the lined tray, shaping it into 6 thin mini pizza bases.
5. Place the tray in the oven and bake for 15–20 minutes, or until the bases are golden and slightly crispy.
6. Remove the bases from the oven, spread tomato passata on each base, sprinkle with cheese, and top with chicken and veggies.
7. Place the pizzas under the grill for 3–5 minutes, or until the cheese is melted and bubbly.

PROTEIN 37 GRAMS, CARBS 30 GRAMS, FAT 15 GRAMS

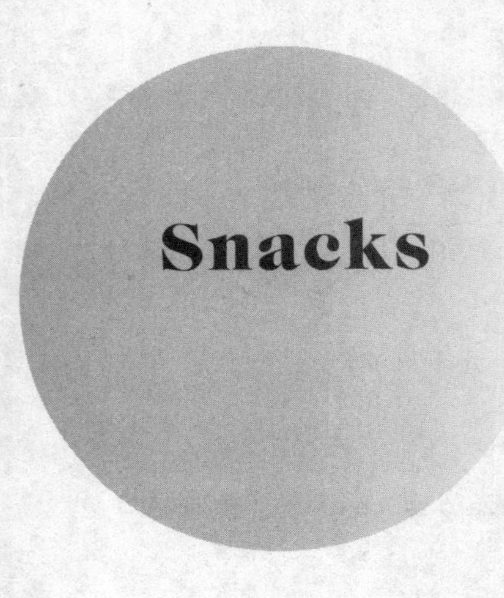

Snacks

Greek Yogurt, Blueberries, and Hemp Seeds

Serves 1

Ingredients

1 tablespoon hemp seeds

⅔ cup plain Greek yogurt

⅓ cup fresh blueberries

Method

1. In a bowl, combine the hemp seeds with the yogurt.
2. Top the yogurt mixture with fresh blueberries and serve.

PROTEIN 17 GRAMS, CARBS 11 GRAMS, FAT 6 GRAMS

Rotisserie Chicken and Hummus Snack Plate

Serves 1

Ingredients

2 ounces rotisserie chicken, shredded

2 tablespoons hummus

4–6 small whole-grain crackers

1 small cucumber, sliced

1 small carrot, sliced into sticks

Method

1. On a plate, arrange the shredded chicken, hummus, crackers, cucumber, and carrot sticks.
2. Enjoy as a light, protein-packed snack.

PROTEIN 16 GRAMS, CARBS 15 GRAMS, FAT 11 GRAMS

Carrot and Salmon Dip

Serves 1

Ingredients

Small can (3.75 ounces) of wild salmon, flaked

3–4 tablespoons plain Greek yogurt

1 tablespoon finely chopped chives

Squeeze of lemon juice

Sea salt and black pepper, to taste

1 medium carrot, peeled and cut into sticks

1 celery stalk, cut into sticks

Method

1. In a bowl, mix the salmon, yogurt, chives, and lemon juice.
2. Season with sea salt and black pepper to taste.
3. Serve the salmon and yogurt dip with the carrot and celery sticks.

PROTEIN 24 GRAMS, CARBS 9 GRAMS, FAT 10 GRAMS

Broccoli and Sweet Potato Egg Muffin

Serves 4 (2 muffins per serving)

Ingredients

1 medium sweet potato, peeled and chopped into cubes

1 medium broccoli head, cut into florets

8 large eggs

½ teaspoon sea salt

½ teaspoon black pepper

Method

1. Preheat the oven to 350°F. Grease a muffin tray or insert cupcake liners.
2. Steam the sweet potato for 10 minutes.
3. Add the broccoli to the steamer and cook for another 5 minutes (with the potatoes). Once the veggies are done, evenly distribute them into the prepared muffin tray.
4. In a mixing bowl, whisk the eggs and season with sea salt and black pepper.
5. Pour the whisked egg mixture into the muffin tray, ensuring the sweet potato and broccoli are evenly covered.
6. Bake for 15–18 minutes, or until the eggs are fully cooked through.
7. Store the egg muffins in the refrigerator for a convenient and nutritious snack.

PROTEIN 15 GRAMS, CARBS 12 GRAMS, FAT 13 GRAMS

Cottage Cheese and Stewed Apples

Serves 1

Ingredients

⅔ cup cottage cheese

½ cup Stewed Apples (page 293)

Method

Serve the cottage cheese with the stewed apples and enjoy!

PROTEIN 18 GRAMS, CARBS 15 GRAMS, FAT 3 GRAMS

Gut-Healing Recipes

Stewed Apples

Ingredients

6 apples, washed, cored, and sliced into even pieces

2 teaspoons ground cinnamon

1 teaspoon pure vanilla extract

Method

1. Place the sliced apples in a saucepan or pot, then add the cinnamon and vanilla extract.
2. Add ½ cup of water to the pan. Turn the heat to medium-high and bring to a simmer. Then reduce the heat to low and cover the saucepan with a lid.
3. Let the apples stew gently for about 10 minutes, or until they are tender but not mushy, stirring occasionally.
4. Once the apples are cooked to your liking, remove them from the heat, and let them cool slightly before serving.
5. Store any leftover stewed apples in an airtight container in the refrigerator for up to 5 days.

Beef Bone Broth

Ingredients

3 pounds beef bones (preferably marrow or knuckle bones)

2 carrots, roughly chopped

2 celery stalks, roughly chopped

1 onion, peeled and quartered

4 garlic cloves, smashed

2 bay leaves

2 tablespoons apple cider vinegar

Method

1. Preheat the oven to 400°F.
2. Place the beef bones on a baking tray and roast in the oven for about 30 minutes, or until they are browned and caramelized.
3. Transfer the roasted bones to a large stockpot or slow cooker.
4. Add the carrots, celery, onion, garlic, bay leaves, and apple cider vinegar to the pot.
5. Fill the pot with enough water to cover the bones completely.
6. Bring the water to the boil over high heat, then reduce the heat to low and let the broth simmer gently for at least 12 hours or for longer (about 24 hours) in a slow cooker or Instant Pot (with a slow-cook function).
7. Once the broth is done simmering, remove it from the heat and let it cool slightly.
8. Strain the broth through a fine-mesh sieve into a clean container.
9. Let the broth cool completely before storing it in the refrigerator or freezer.

Chicken Bone Broth

Ingredients

3 pounds chicken bones (backs, necks, or carcasses)

2 carrots, roughly chopped

2 celery stalks, roughly chopped

1 onion, peeled and quartered

4 garlic cloves, smashed

2 bay leaves

2 tablespoons apple cider vinegar

Method

1. Preheat the oven to 400°F.
2. Place the chicken bones on a baking sheet and roast them in the oven for about 30 minutes, or until they are browned and caramelized.
3. Transfer the roasted bones to a large stockpot or slow cooker.
4. Add the carrots, celery, onion, garlic, bay leaves, and apple cider vinegar to the pot.
5. Fill the pot with enough water to cover the bones completely.
6. Bring the water to a boil over high heat, then reduce the heat to low and let the broth simmer gently for at least 6–8 hours, or for longer (about 18 hours) in a slow cooker or Instant Pot (with a slow-cook function).
7. Once the broth is done simmering, remove it from the heat and let it cool slightly.
8. Strain the broth through a fine-mesh sieve into a clean container.
9. Let the broth cool completely before storing it in the refrigerator or freezer.

Homemade Sauerkraut

Ingredients

1 medium (about 2 pounds) green cabbage, finely shredded (the thinner the better)

3–4 teaspoons sea salt (1.5–2 percent of cabbage weight), plus more for extra brine as needed

Method

1. Sterilize a 1-quart glass jar and a mixing bowl by pouring boiling water over them to ensure they're clean.
2. Add the cabbage to the mixing bowl and sprinkle with the salt.
3. Knead and squeeze the cabbage for a few minutes until it begins releasing liquid.
4. Cover the bowl and let it rest, returning every 10 minutes to knead and squeeze again. Repeat until enough liquid forms to fully cover the cabbage when pressed down.
5. Transfer the cabbage and its liquid into the sterilized jar, pressing it down firmly so it's completely submerged in the liquid.
6. Use a fermentation weight to keep the cabbage fully submerged. If there isn't enough liquid to cover the cabbage by at least ½ inch, make extra brine by dissolving 1 teaspoon of sea salt in 1 cup of filtered water and pour just enough over the cabbage to submerge it.
7. Cover with a fermentation lid with a built-in airlock. Store in a cool, dark place (65–72°F) for 1–2 weeks. The warmer it is, the quicker it will ferment, so be mindful in the summer months.
8. Check regularly, pressing down the weight if needed to keep the cabbage submerged. If you see any exposed cabbage, push it back under the brine.
9. Taste after a week—it's ready when it reaches your preferred level of tanginess (typically around 10 days).
10. Once ready, seal the jar and transfer it to the fridge. It can last for up to 6 months as long as you use a clean utensil every time you use it.

Ginger Water

Ingredients

1 inch fresh ginger root (no need to peel if organic)

Juice of ½ lemon (optional)

Method

1. Rinse the ginger root under cold water to remove any dirt.
2. Slice the ginger and place it in a blender. Add 1–2 cups water, depending on how strong you want the ginger flavor to be.
3. Blend the ginger and water at high speed for about 30 seconds.
4. Place a fine-mesh sieve or cheesecloth over a clean container. Pour the blended ginger water through the sieve or cheesecloth to strain out the ginger pulp. Use a spoon to press down on the ginger pulp to extract as much liquid as possible.
5. Transfer the strained ginger water to a glass or bottle for storage. You can enjoy ginger water immediately or refrigerate it for 2 or 3 days.
6. Optional: Stir in the lemon juice just before serving.

Moving Forward

Life Beyond the Plan

As we come to the end of this book, I invite you to think about the bigger picture—how to make the Cortisol Reset Plan a lasting part of your life.

We've worked through a powerful plan—one that nurtures both your body and mind, with a particular focus on balancing your cortisol levels. Cortisol is a crucial indicator of how well your body adapts to stress, influencing everything from energy and immune function to metabolism and sleep. When cortisol levels are balanced—neither too high nor too low—your body is better equipped to achieve the overarching goal we set at the start of this book: a strong body and a calm mind.

Here's a recap of what we've covered:

- **Step One:** We started by focusing on nourishing your body with unprocessed, whole, nutrient-dense foods that provide the fuel needed to produce energy, improve resilience, and enhance your ability to manage stress.

- **Step Two:** Next, we explored how stabilizing your blood sugar helps maintain steady energy levels, supports hormonal balance, and reduces stress.
- **Step Three:** We then aligned your daily activities with your body's natural circadian rhythm, with a special focus on mastering light exposure, as well as meal timing and exercise, to support improved energy, mood, and sleep quality.
- **Step Four:** We incorporated exercise, designed to challenge and support your body, helping to reduce stress and boost overall resilience.
- **Step Five:** Finally, we worked on cultivating psychological resilience, using tools and practices that improve emotional regulation and stress management, empowering you to navigate life's challenges with greater calm and confidence. Only when the body feels safe and settled can we begin to do this deeper mental and spiritual work that leads to true healing.

The true transformation comes when you begin integrating these practices into your everyday routine—slowly, steadily, and with compassion, for the long term. The key to lasting change is consistently incorporating at least one habit from each of the steps every day. Some days will feel easy, and you might find yourself able to do a few things from each step. On other days, it will feel more challenging, but these are the days when committing to at least one action from each step will make the most difference.

Let me give you an example of how you can achieve one

thing from each step on a challenging day when you have very little time: Start your day with one of the breakfast options in Part III—pages 263–69 (Steps One and Two, checked). Then, go for a brisk 15-minute walk after breakfast (Steps Three and Four, checked). Finally, take a few minutes in the middle of your day to check in with your body sensations and take a few deep breaths to reset (Step Five, checked). At the end of each day, assess how it went. Were you able to achieve one thing from each step? If so, amazing—celebrate your efforts! If not, give yourself compassion and try again tomorrow. Remember, it's the small, consistent actions that add up over time. Little by little, you'll be amazed at the progress you make when you focus on just one step each day.

Let this book be a road map you can return to whenever you need. Embrace the journey, learn from each of the steps, and always trust in your limitless potential.

Some closing reminders

- The healing journey isn't linear, and that's okay. There will be days and weeks of progress, plateaus, and setbacks. The important thing is the overall pattern over time. Sometimes, you may need to take a step back before moving forward. Don't let that disappoint you; it's just a normal part of the process.
- You are already enough. While you have the potential to learn and grow, remember that you don't need to be anyone else to be worthy of love. Compassion and kindness toward yourself should always be your compass on this journey.
- One small habit is all you need to start, followed by another, and then another. This is not a sprint—you have a lifetime to refine your skills and reach your full potential.

- You are not alone. Even when you feel isolated in your struggles, remember that challenges are an inherent part of the human experience. This is how we grow, and we can all do it together.
- Always challenge your thoughts. Remember, you are not your thoughts; you are the observing Self, the one listening to them. Be curious, question their truth, and learn to observe them without identifying with them.

Acknowledgments

My shift from a high-pressure corporate career to holistic health was a professional change and a big personal transformation. But I never in a million years imagined this journey would lead me to write a book!

I am deeply grateful to everyone who has contributed to bringing this project to life, directly, and indirectly. As the saying goes, a book is not solely the work of the person on the cover; it takes a dedicated team of incredible people to turn an idea into reality.

First and foremost, I extend my heartfelt appreciation to my editors in the United Kingdom, Anya Hayes and Julia Kellaway. Your belief in me and this project planted a seed that has blossomed into reality. Thank you immensely. I would not be here without your support and guidance.

A big shout-out to the entire team at Ebury and PRH, including Marta Catalano and Kate Latham for your amazing work refining the manuscript and making sure everything is clear and polished, and to Sarah Scarlett, Ann-Katrin Ziser, Penelope Liechti, Monique Corless, and Elizabeth Brandon, for your incredible work on making this book accessible to readers in numerous countries. I know many more people are working behind the scenes, and I sincerely appreciate every single one of you.

I also want to thank my US publisher, HarperOne, and my editor Nina Shield, along with her team, including Daphney Guillaume, Crissie Molina, and Hope Clarke. Your insights and attention to detail have been invaluable in shaping and bringing this book to its fullest potential.

My clients and students have shaped the foundations of the Cortisol Reset Plan. Their experiences keep contributing to my learning and personal growth. I deeply appreciate your trust in sharing your health journeys with me.

To my mentors and colleagues who have generously shared their knowledge and expertise, as well as the brilliant scientists and researchers whose work has inspired my passion for science and contributed to shaping my understanding and refining my ideas—I am very grateful for your dedication and hard work, and I've strived to do justice to your contributions throughout this book.

A heartfelt thank-you to my dearest friends, Ana María García, Sarah Sutherland, and Emma Steven, for our long phone calls, walks, coffee breaks, and countless shared moments.

My family remains my backbone. Thanks to my father and my brothers for your love and encouragement, and to my husband's family for welcoming me as one of your own.

To my children, Oscar and Bas—you are my best teachers. Becoming a mum has changed me in ways I never expected. You've shown me what unconditional love really means, and every day with you reminds me how deep that love goes.

Lastly, and most importantly, to my husband, Max. Your mere presence regulates my nervous system! Thank you for your patience during the long hours of this project and for creating the space and encouragement I need to pursue personal and professional growth.

Appendix A

At-Home Cortisol Testing

Cortisol can be measured in blood, urine, saliva, or a combination of these. My preference is for urine or saliva, and I recommend a diurnal (four-point) cortisol test.

Cortisol levels naturally fluctuate throughout the day in a pattern known as the "diurnal rhythm." A four-point test captures these fluctuations, allowing for a better understanding of how cortisol levels change over a 24-hour period. In contrast, a single-point test provides only a snapshot of cortisol levels at one point in time, which may not accurately represent the overall cortisol rhythm.

Here are two tests and labs I routinely recommend for my clients, which you can also order yourself:

1. Dried Urine Test for Comprehensive Hormones (DUTCH). There are three options, depending on your budget/needs:

DUTCH Adrenal

- Focuses on cortisol, cortisone, their metabolites, and DHEA-S.

- Ideal for people primarily looking to assess adrenal function and stress response.

DUTCH Complete

- More comprehensive than the DUTCH Adrenal.
- Includes a full profile of sex hormones (estrogen, progesterone, testosterone) and adrenal hormones (including cortisol, DHEA-S, and their metabolites), as well as melatonin and oxidative stress markers.
- Provides a thorough picture of overall hormonal health, helping to identify hormonal imbalances.

DUTCH Plus

- The most expensive and detailed.
- Includes everything from the DUTCH Complete, plus the Cortisol Awakening Response (CAR) for deeper insight into HPA axis function.
- Great for advanced assessment of cortisol and hormonal patterns but may not be necessary unless there's a specific need for a deeper dive.

2. Adrenal Stress Profile by ZRT Laboratory

Appendix B

Ways to Reduce Your Toxin Exposure

Environmental toxins add to the "wear and tear" on your body, reducing your resilience to stress and disease through various mechanisms, including increasing inflammation, disrupting mitochondrial function (which impairs your body's ability to produce energy efficiently), interfering with hormonal signaling, altering feedback mechanisms that hinder homeostasis, and elevating oxidative stress, among others.

These are invisible and "fly under our radar," but they are chronic stressors that quietly add to your "stress bucket." The good news? With a few simple swaps, you can significantly limit your exposure.

The first step is awareness. You need to know where these toxins are:

- **Pesticides:** Many pesticides, including atrazine and organophosphate pesticides, disrupt the endocrine system. They are used in agriculture to control weeds and pests on crops, and they pose risks to human health through dietary exposure and environmental contamination.[1] You can find pesticides in conventionally grown fruits, vegetables, grains, and contaminated water sources near agricultural areas.

- **Phthalates:** Phthalates are used to make plastics more flexible and are also found as stabilizers in fragrances. These chemicals can interfere with hormone function and have been associated with reproductive problems, respiratory issues, and developmental abnormalities.[2] Phthalates are commonly found in plastic products such as food containers, shower curtains, and vinyl flooring, as well as in personal care products like cosmetics, fragrances, and nail polish.
- **Parabens:** Used as preservatives in various food and personal care products, parabens have been shown to disrupt hormone activity in the body.[3] Parabens can be found in a wide range of products, including cosmetics, lotions, shampoos, and processed foods.
- **Perchlorate:** Perchlorate is used in rocket propellants, munitions, fireworks, and other products, and it can contaminate food and water sources. Exposure to perchlorate can disrupt thyroid function, affecting metabolism and overall health.[4] Perchlorate contamination is often found in drinking water sources near military bases, industrial sites, and areas with extensive fireworks displays.
- **Heavy metals:** Certain heavy metals, such as lead, mercury, and cadmium, can act as endocrine disruptors when they accumulate in the body.[5] They are found in various consumer products, industrial processes, and contaminated food and

water sources. Heavy metals can be present in lead-based paints, seafood, and industrial runoff in waterways.

- **Perfluoroalkyl and polyfluoroalkyl substances (PFAS):** Also known as "forever chemicals," PFAS are commonly used in products to make them resistant to heat, oil, stains, and water. These chemicals have been linked to hormonal disruptions, reproductive issues, and an increased risk of cancer.[6] PFAS can be found in nonstick cookware, waterproof clothing, food packaging, and firefighting foam used at airports and military bases.

- **Bisphenol A (BPA) and BPA alternatives:** BPA is found in some canned foods, thermal paper (receipts), and plastic products. Exposure to BPA and its alternatives has been associated with various health problems, including hormonal imbalances, reproductive issues, and cancer.[7]

- **Oxybenzone:** Oxybenzone is a UV filter found in sunscreens and SPF products. Research suggests that oxybenzone can interfere with the endocrine system and may increase the risk of adverse birth outcomes and certain cancers.[8] Oxybenzone is present in many sunscreens, lip balms, and moisturizers with SPF protection.

Now, let's make a few simple changes to reduce your exposure. I've grouped them into a few categories to keep it simple: food and water, kitchen, personal care, and home.

You don't need to make all the changes at once, so please don't feel overwhelmed. Also, unlike the habits you've adopted in the five steps of the Cortisol Reset Plan, most of the changes you're going to make here aren't daily habits you need to maintain. Instead, they're one-time actions with long-term benefits. For example, replacing your plastic food containers with glass ones is a one-off change that can significantly reduce your exposure to hormone-disrupting chemicals over time.

Start with Your Food and Water

A big portion of the environmental toxins we encounter daily comes from the food we eat and the water we drink. But don't worry, you can limit your exposure in a few manageable stages.

PACKAGED FOODS

It is unrealistic to avoid packaged foods completely, but my simple rule is to choose products with a *minimal* number of ingredients that you can easily understand. A lengthy list of ingredients or ingredients that you don't understand should raise a red flag.

For instance, when buying yogurt, look for straightforward ingredients like milk and live cultures. If you come across a yogurt with a long ingredient list such as "water, sugar, fructose, modified corn starch, carob bean gum, lactic acid, and sodium citrate," it's best to pass on it.

FRESH FRUITS AND VEGETABLES

When it comes to fruits and vegetables, organic or biodynamic is ideal. Choosing organic means selecting non-GMO (genetically modified organism) items grown without synthetic pesticides and fertilizers. These are grown using traditional methods and avoiding genetic modifications that may have unknown long-term effects on human health and the environment.

Now, I know that organic is a lot more expensive, but fortunately, you don't necessarily need to buy everything organic. Some particular fruits and vegetables have been shown to contain worrisome amounts of pesticides, such as strawberries. However, there are plenty of conventional produce items that are reasonably safe. This means that you can be selective and save your money for what really matters. The Dirty Dozen and Clean Fifteen are lists published annually by the Environmental Working Group (EWG) that aim to guide consumers in making informed choices about purchasing fruits and vegetables based on their pesticide exposure.[9]

Thoroughly washing produce can also significantly reduce pesticide residues. Even organic produce and prewashed bagged salad should be rinsed to remove any remaining handling residues. For nonorganic produce, peeling the outer layers (when possible) can further minimize exposure to pesticides.

ANIMAL PRODUCTS

When choosing animal-based products such as meat, dairy, fish, and other seafood, try to prioritize the best quality you can afford:

- For beef and dairy, choose grass-fed. Organic products are the next best choice.
- For poultry and eggs, seek out products from farms that raise pastured birds. The second best is organic poultry and eggs that come from birds raised without the use of antibiotics, hormones, synthetic pesticides, or GMOs. Free range is the third best option.
- For fish, prioritize wild-caught varieties over farmed options, and look for fish low in mercury, a toxic heavy metal

that tends to accumulate in larger fish such as bigeye tuna (canned tuna, especially skipjack tuna, has lower levels), swordfish, king mackerel, shark, swordfish, and barramundi. Opt for fish with lower mercury levels, such as salmon, sardines, trout, and mackerel.

WATER

One of the best ways to reduce your exposure to toxins is by using a good water filter. Water can contain heavy metals, pesticides, industrial chemicals, and microbial pathogens. One recent global study showed that disinfection by-products commonly found in tap water can negatively impact fertility and reproductive health.[10] Since you drink water constantly, investing in a water filter is one of the best decisions you can make for your long-term health.

Now that we have addressed the food you eat and the water you drink, let's move on to the next step: tackling environmental toxins in the kitchen.

Create a Toxin-Free Kitchen Environment

Let me show you a few simple swaps in your kitchen that will greatly decrease your exposure risk from cookware, food storage containers, chopping boards, kitchen utensils, and cleaning products.

COOKWARE

In recent years, there has been a growing awareness of the potential health risks associated with nonstick coatings. These coatings often contain perfluorinated chemicals (PFCs), including perfluorooctanoic acid and other PFAS. PFCs have raised concerns about their ability to leach into food, especially under high temperatures during cooking. My recommendation is to ditch your nonstick cookware and replace it with the following:

- stainless steel
- cast iron
- enameled cast iron
- carbon steel
- glass
- pure ceramic

FOOD STORAGE CONTAINERS

Plastics harbor bisphenols A, S, and F, as well as polychlorinated biphenyls. To reduce your exposure to plastics, consider the following swaps:

- Replace disposable plastic bottles with stainless steel.
- Substitute plastic wraps with eco-friendly beeswax wraps.
- Opt for glass instead of plastic containers for storing leftovers and meal prepping. You can also use mason jars for storing pantry items, liquids or prepped meals.
- Minimize your reliance on canned foods, even those labelled BPA-free. Instead, opt for frozen, Tetra Pak, or glass-packaged alternatives.

- Replace single-use plastic bags with reusable silicone food storage bags.
- Instead of plastic lunch containers, switch to stainless steel lunchboxes.

CUTTING BOARDS

In a study featured in the journal *Environmental Science & Technology*, researchers showed the presence of microplastics in food following the use of plastic cutting boards.[11] To reduce your plastic exposure, consider one of these safer options instead:

- Cutting boards made from natural wood, particularly hardwoods like maple, walnut, and cherry.
- Epicurean cutting boards. While epicurean is generally nontoxic, ensure it is UL GREENGUARD Certified.
- Cutting boards made from 100 percent high-density natural rubber.

KITCHEN UTENSILS

The next step is to consider the quality of your kitchen utensils. We use our utensils every day and they come into direct contact with our food, so here are your best options:

- wooden utensils, like bamboo, beech, or maple wood
- stainless steel
- silicone

CLEANING PRODUCTS

Look for brands that specialize in eco-friendly cleaners, but be cautious about marketing gimmicks when buying "green" or "nontoxic" products. Check for certifications such as the Environmental Protection Agency's Safer Choice, Green Seal, or ECOLOGO. Try to avoid products that contain the following ingredients: phthalates, sulphates such as sodium lauryl sulphate and sodium laureth sulphate, triclosan, quaternary ammonium compounds, 2-butoxyethanol, ammonia, chlorine, and sodium hydroxide.

Alternatively, if you like the idea of making your own cleaning products, the following recipes are 100 percent safe and cost-effective! You probably already have most of the ingredients you need in your home:

- baking soda
- borax
- coarse salt
- coconut oil (fractionated)
- essential oils: tea tree, lemon, or lavender
- lemon
- liquid castile soap
- olive oil
- rubbing alcohol
- vegetable glycerin
- vinegar
- washing soda (sodium carbonate)

All-purpose cleaner: Mix 1 cup white vinegar with 1 cup water in a 16-ounce spray bottle. Optionally, add 10 to 15 drops of essential oil. Shake well to combine the ingredients.

Window and glass cleaner: Mix ½ cup white vinegar with ½ cup rubbing alcohol and put in a 16-ounce spray bottle; fill the rest with water.

All-purpose floor cleaner: Mix 1 cup white vinegar with 1 gallon warm water in a bucket. Optionally, add a few drops of essential oil.

Wood polish: Combine ½ cup olive oil, ½ cup white vinegar, 1 tablespoon vegetable glycerin, and 1 teaspoon coconut oil in a bowl. Optionally, add a few drops of essential oil.

Cleaner for wooden chopping boards: Cut a lemon in half; add coarse salt to the chopping board. Use the lemon halves to scrub the board, pressing to release the juice. Let the mixture sit for a few minutes, then rinse the board with water.

Laundry liquid: Dissolve 1 cup baking soda and 1 cup borax in 1 quart boiling water, stirring until fully dissolved. Remove from the heat and add 1 cup liquid castile soap, stirring to combine. Then, add 2 more quarts water, mixing gently. Allow the solution to cool, then transfer it to an airtight container. For each load, use about ⅓ cup detergent.

Prioritize Safe Choices in Personal Care

It's time to turn our attention to the bathroom because, unfortunately, many of the ingredients in beauty products aren't pretty. Here are three simple tips:

1. GET RID OF FRAGRANCES

If you only make one change, eliminating fragrances will give you the biggest bang for your buck. There's no need to ditch all your fragranced products. Instead, make it a habit to check the label when you purchase a new product. If you spot "fragrance," "perfume," or "parfum," put it back and consider opting for a fragrance-free alternative.

2. SIMPLIFY YOUR ROUTINE

A consumer survey by the EWG found that women use an average of 12 personal care products daily, totaling 168 different chemicals, and adolescent girls use 17.[12] Here's my suggestion: Lay out all the products you currently use. Do you genuinely need every single one? Take a moment to find the ones you don't need—*and stop using them.* As for the products you know you need, consider replacing them with better options when they run out.

3. FIND NONTOXIC PRODUCTS

Get into the habit of scrutinizing labels. Here is a list of common chemicals frequently flagged by researchers and consumer advocacy groups:

- **Parabens:** Found in shampoos, conditioners, lotions, facial cleansers, deodorants, toothpaste, and makeup.
- **Phthalates:** Found in synthetic fragrance, hairspray, nail polish, makeup, shampoo, conditioner, facial cream, and lotions.
- **Butylated hydroxyanisole:** Found in lipsticks, eyeliners, moisturizers, and other products containing oils or fats.

- **Coal tar dyes (for example, m-, o-, and p-phenylenediamine):** Found in hair dyes.
- **Diethanolamine:** Found in shampoos, shaving creams, and other creamy or foamy products.
- **Formaldehyde and formaldehyde releasers:** Found in soaps, body washes, shampoos, liquid baby soaps, and nail polishes.
- **Isobutane, propane, and other propellants:** Found in aerosol sprays like dry shampoos, sunscreens, and deodorants.
- **Polyethylene glycols:** Found in liquid hand soaps, makeup, and creams.
- **Talc:** Found in cosmetics and body powders.
- **Toluene:** Found in nail products and hair dyes.
- **Triclosan and triclocarban:** Formerly found in soaps and still found in toothpaste.
- **1,4-dioxane:** Found in shampoos, soaps, and other products that get sudsy or foamy.
- **Heavy metals (for example, aluminum, lead, cadmium, nickel, and mercury):** Found in lightening creams, cosmetics containing natural minerals and dyes, and deodorant.
- **Perfluorinated chemicals:** Found in anti-ageing products.
- **P-phenylenediamine:** Found in hair dye.
- **Hydroquinone:** Found in skin lightening and brightening products.

- **Titanium dioxide (nanoparticle):** Found in sunscreen and cosmetics with sun protection.
- **Ammonia:** Found in hair dye.
- **Petroleum and petrolatum:** Found in lotions and cosmetics.

One reliable resource is the EWG's Skin Deep database, which offers comprehensive information about the ingredients in various skincare, cosmetic, and personal care products, along with their potential health effects. You can search for specific products or ingredients to evaluate their safety ratings. They also provide a score based on the number of hazards linked to various chemicals. Clearya's browser extension and the Campaign for Safe Cosmetics' Non-Toxic Black Beauty Database have similar offerings.

The MADE SAFE website allows you to search for certified products. Products that meet their criteria receive the MADE SAFE seal, indicating that they are free from a range of potentially harmful ingredients.

Another option is safecosmetics.org, operated by the Campaign for Safe Cosmetics, a project by Breast Cancer Prevention Partners. This website provides a wealth of information about the chemicals to avoid in your personal care products, helping you to make informed choices.

Cultivate a Green Living Space

According to the Environmental Protection Agency, indoor air can be more heavily polluted than outdoor air, even in the largest and most industrialized cities.[13] The pollutants come from air fresheners, candles, cleaning products, paints, varnishes, furniture, pesticides, building materials, fireplaces, and gas stoves. Additionally, factors such as inadequate ventilation, dust, and mold can further contribute to indoor air pollution.

The following four steps will greatly improve your indoor air quality:

1. OPEN THE WINDOWS

The simplest and most effective way to improve the air in your home is to open the doors and windows often. This allows fresh outdoor air to come in, getting rid of stale air. It helps to decrease indoor pollutants, including volatile organic compounds, mold spores, and other harmful pollutants. Depending on the weather, try to keep your windows open for as much of the day as possible.

If opening windows regularly isn't possible, another effective way to improve indoor air quality is by using air filters. In particular, high-efficiency particulate air (HEPA) filters are well-known for their ability to get rid of a wide range of airborne particles, including dust, pollen, pet dander, mold spores, and even bacteria and viruses.

2. GET INDOOR PLANTS

There are a few plants that can help filter out toxic chemicals from the air:*

- aloe vera (*Aloe barbadensis*)
- areca palm (*Dypsis lutescens*)
- bamboo palm (*Chamaedorea seifrizii*)

* If you have a pet, make sure to choose pet-friendly options, as some plants can be harmful to animals.

- Boston fern (*Nephrolepis exaltata*)
- dracaena (*Dracaena* spp.)
- English ivy (*Hedera helix*)
- peace lily (*Spathiphyllum* spp.)
- rubber plant (*Ficus elastica*)
- snake plant (*Sansevieria trifasciata*)
- spider plant (*Chlorophytum comosum*)

3. ATTACK THE DUST

You won't be able to eliminate all dust in your home, but you can reduce it with these three steps:

1. **Leave your shoes at the door:** Stop tracking outdoor contaminants indoors by adopting the habit of leaving your shoes at the door.
2. **Vacuum regularly:** Vacuum often to capture dust particles and other contaminants. A vacuum with a HEPA filter will be the most effective at this.
3. **Wet mop your house:** Instead of relying solely on a traditional broom, use a wet mop. Wet mopping traps and removes more dust particles.

4. DITCH THE SCENTED CANDLES AND AIR FRESHENERS

Any product designed to release artificial scents into the air is likely to contain chemicals such as phthalates, and they can release volatile organic compounds. Candles also often contain paraffin wax, a petroleum-derived substance that releases harmful chemicals when burned. The best and safest way to get a fresh smell in your house is to open the windows and get that ventilation going.

You now have the tools you need to effectively decrease your stress load by minimizing your toxin exposure from your surroundings. As I said at the start, you don't have to make too many changes all at once. Think of this section as an ongoing process to slowly and progressively decrease your exposure to toxins over the next few weeks and months.

Appendix C

Consider Adaptogens and Other Nutritional Compounds

Let's now dive into the world of adaptogenic herbs, often simply referred to as "adaptogens," as well as other nutritional compounds that have the ability to enhance your resilience to stress.

Adaptogens

Adaptogens are a class of botanicals, primarily derived from plants, that can help the body adapt to stressors, whether physical or emotional. Named by Russian scientist Dr. Nikolai Lazarev in the 1950s, adaptogens can increase "the state of non-specific resistance" in stress, which means they might improve the body's resilience to various stressors.[1]

Research shows that adaptogens have multiple beneficial effects, including reducing fatigue, decreasing symptoms of depression and anxiety, and improving cognitive function (nootropic effects). While the exact mechanisms are not fully understood, studies suggest that, at a molecular level, adaptogens might help regulate homeostasis, interact with the HPA axis, and influence the stress response through mediators like cortisol.[2]

In *Adaptogens: Herbs for Strength, Stamina, and Stress Relief*, herbalist David Winston and researcher Steven Maimes offer an extensive exploration of adaptogens and present a wealth of knowledge that encompasses various adaptogenic herbs and their benefits, plus dosages and cautions.[3] Drawing from their expertise, I will discuss five adaptogens with a long history of safety.

If you want to try an adaptogen, please check with your doctor first to make sure it is appropriate for you. Also, before choosing an adaptogen, check the results of your questionnaires in "How the Cortisol Reset Plan Will Help You Thrive" (pages 47–50) and choose the one that aligns most closely with your symptoms and your needs.

ASHWAGANDHA (*WITHANIA SOMNIFERA*)

Originating from traditional Ayurvedic medicine, ashwagandha is one of the most studied adaptogens and is known for its ability to reduce stress and anxiety.

A double-blinded RCT found that it "safely and effectively improves an individual's resistance towards stress and thereby improves self-assessed quality of life."[4] A review of five clinical trials showed a statistical improvement in anxiety or stress measurements with this adaptogen.[5] Another RCT suggested that ashwagandha root can also stimulate the thyroid, making it useful for mild cases of hypothyroidism.[6]

Best for: Anxiety or feelings of nervousness, fatigue, brain fog, and insomnia.

Dosage: One 300–500 milligram capsule, twice per day.

Safety issues: Avoid using this herb if you are sensitive to plants in the nightshade family (see page 101) or you have hyperthyroid disease. There are no human studies to confirm its safety during pregnancy and breastfeeding.

RHODIOLA (*RHODIOLA ROSEA*)

From the mountainous regions of Europe and Asia, rhodiola is known for its energy-boosting properties and its capacity to enhance endurance and resilience in the face of stress.

Rhodiola is a stimulating adaptogen that can enhance alertness, reduce fatigue, improve memory, and relieve depression. A review of 11 RCTs showed that it can have beneficial effects on physical performance, depression, mild anxiety, and overall mood.[7]

Best for: Brain fog, anxiety and depression, poor exercise tolerance, and physical fatigue/exhaustion.

Dosage: 200–600 milligrams per day may be effective (in divided doses).

Safety issues: Avoid taking before bedtime as it has a slightly stimulating effect. There are no human studies to confirm its safety during pregnancy and breastfeeding.

ASIAN GINSENG (*PANAX GINSENG*)

Known as the "king of herbs" in traditional Chinese medicine, *Panax ginseng* is considered to be the most stimulating of all adaptogens, known for its ability to improve energy levels and cognitive function.

A review of 10 studies concluded that ginseng could significantly improve fatigue.[8] Other studies show it can improve mood and memory,[9] and it may offer benefits for depression and anxiety.[10]

Best for: Exhaustion and poor memory.

Dosage: 200–400 milligrams daily.

Safety issues: There are no human studies to confirm its safety during pregnancy and breastfeeding.

HOLY BASIL (*OCIMUM SANCTUM*)

Also known as tulsi, holy basil is a nourishing adaptogen with antioxidant properties. A review of 24 studies showed that tulsi was effective in improving mood, cognitive function, and relieving anxiety and perceived stress levels.[11]

Best for: Anxiety, sleep problems, inflammation, and high blood sugar.

Dosage: 300–2,000 milligrams daily.

Safety issues: Avoid in pregnancy or when trying to conceive.

Other Botanicals and Nutritional Compounds

Lastly, here are two botanicals that aren't classified as adaptogens, but can be helpful in balancing cortisol levels when they are either too high or too low.

PHOSPHATIDYLSERINE (FOR HIGH CORTISOL)

Phosphatidylserine (PS) is a phospholipid found in the brain that is crucial for maintaining brain structure and function, such as supporting memory. It can be found in food such as organ meats, fish, or egg yolks, or in supplement form.

Interestingly, PS has been studied for its role in reducing cortisol levels and blunting the body's stress response, which makes it beneficial for those of you who scored highly on the high cortisol questionnaire on page 47.[12]

> **Dosage:** Around 200–300 milligrams per day (in divided doses) have shown beneficial effects.[13]

LICORICE ROOT (FOR LOW CORTISOL)

The key component of licorice root, glycyrrhizin, has been shown to inhibit the enzyme responsible for converting cortisol into its inactive form, cortisone. This means that it extends the life of cortisol, leading to higher cortisol levels.[14] This can be helpful for those of you who scored highly on the low cortisol questionnaire on page 49.

However, licorice root carries certain risks, particularly the potential to raise blood pressure. Therefore, it should be taken with caution and is only for short-term use. It is especially important to avoid licorice root if you have high blood pressure. Additionally, excessive or prolonged use of licorice root can lead to other side effects such as electrolyte imbalances and potassium depletion. Always consult with a healthcare provider before starting licorice root supplementation, since appropriate dosing and monitoring are key.

Notes

Understanding the Nervous System

1. Jane Ogden, *Health Psychology: A Textbook*, 3rd ed. (Open Univ. Press, 2004), 259.
2. Bruce S. McEwen and Peter J. Gianaros, "Stress- and Allostasis-Induced Brain Plasticity," *Annual Review of Medicine*, 62 (2011): 431–45, https://doi.org/10.1146/annurev-med-052209–100430.
3. Walter B. Cannon, *The Wisdom of the Body* (W. W. Norton, 1932), 177–201.
4. Bruce S. McEwen and Eliot Stellar, "Stress and the Individual: Mechanisms Leading to Disease," *Archives of Internal Medicine* 153, no. 18 (1993): 2093–101, https://doi.org/ 10.1001/archinte.1993 .00410180039004.
5. Bruce S. McEwen, "Allostasis, Allostatic Load, and the Aging Nervous System: Role of Excitatory Amino Acids and Excitotoxicity," *Neurochemical Research* 25 (2000): 1219–31 (2000), https://doi.org /10.1023/A:1007687911139.
6. Natalia Bobba-Alves, Robert-Paul Juster, and Martin Picard, "The Energetic Cost of Allostasis and Allostatic Load," *Psychoneuroendocrinology* 146 (2022):105951, https://doi.org/10.1016 /j.psyneuen.2022.105951; Bruce S. McEwen and Peter J. Gianaros, "Stress- and Allostasis-Induced Brain Plasticity," *Annual Review of Medicine* 62 (2011): 431–45, https://doi.org/10.1146/annurev-med -052209–100430.
7. Natalia Bobba-Alves, Robert-Paul Juster, and Martin Picard, "The Energetic Cost of Allostasis and Allostatic Load," *Psychoneuroendocrinology* 146 (2022): 105951, https://doi.org/10.1016 /j.psyneuen.2022.105951.
8. Jenny Guidi, Marcella Lucente, Nicoletta Sonino, and Giovanni A. Fava, "Allostatic Load and Its Impact on Health: A Systematic Review,"

Psychother Psychosom 90, no. 1 (2021): 11–27, https://doi.org/10.1159/000510696.

9. Peter C. Konturek, T. Brzozowski, and S. J. Konturek, "Stress and the Gut: Pathophysiology, Clinical Consequences, Diagnostic Approach and Treatment Options," *Journal of Physiology and Pharmacology* 62, no. 6 (2011): 591–99.
10. Eva Fries, Judith Hesse, Juliane Hellhammer, and Dirk H. Hellhammer, "A New View on Hypocortisolism," *Psychoneuroendocrinology* 30, no. 10 (2005): 1010–16, https://doi.org/10.1016/j.psyneuen.2005.04.006.
11. Nia Fogelman and Turhan Canli, "Early Life Stress and Cortisol: A Meta-Analysis," *Hormones and Behavior* 98 (2018): 63–76, https://doi.org/10.1016/j.yhbeh.2017.12.014.
12. R. M. M. Schoorlemmer, G. M. E. E. Peeters, N. M. Van Schoor, and P. Lips, "Relationships Between Cortisol Level, Mortality and Chronic Diseases in Older Persons," *Clinical Endocrinology* 71, no. 6 (2009): 779–86, https://doi.org/10.1111/j.1365–2265.2009.03552.x.
13. Eva Fries, Judith Hesse, Juliane Hellhammer, and Dirk H. Hellhammer, "A New View on Hypocortisolism," *Psychoneuroendocrinology* 30, no. 10 (2005): 1010–16, https://doi.org/10.1016/j.psyneuen.2005.04.006.

The Four Types of Stressors

1. Thomas Guilliams, *The Role of Stress and the HPA Axis in Chronic Disease Management*, 2nd ed. (Point Institute, 2015).
2. Steven F. Maier and Linda R. Watkins, "Stressor Controllability and Learned Helplessness: The Roles of the Dorsal Raphe Nucleus, Serotonin, and Corticotropin-Releasing Factor," *Neuroscience & Biobehavioral Reviews* 29, no. 4–5 (2005): 829–41, https://doi.org/10.1016/j.neubiorev.2005.03.021.
3. Bruce S. McEwen and Peter J. Gianaros, "Stress- and Allostasis-Induced Brain Plasticity," *Annual Review of Medicine* 62 (2011): 431–45, https://doi.org/10.1146/annurev-med-052209–100430.
4. Rebecca C. Thurston, Mary Y. Carson, Karestan C. Koenen, Yuefang Chang, Karen A. Matthews, Roland von Känel, and J. Richard Jennings, "The Relationship of Trauma Exposure to Heart Rate Variability During Wake and Sleep in Midlife Women," *Psychophysiology* 57, no. 4 (2020): e13514, https://doi.org/10.1111/psyp.13514.
5. Hye-Geum Kim, Eun-Jin Cheon, Dai-Seg Bai, Young Hwan Lee, and Bon-Hoon Koo, "Stress and Heart Rate Variability: A Meta-Analysis and Review of the Literature," *Psychiatry Investigation* 15, no.3 (2018): 235–45, https://doi.org/10.30773/pi.2017.08.17.

6. Victoria P. Belancio, David E. Blask, Prescott Deininger, Steven M. Hill, and S. Michal Jazwinski, "The Aging Clock and Circadian Control of Metabolism and Genome Stability," *Frontiers in Genetics* 5 (2015): 455, https://doi.org/10.3389/fgene.2014.00455.
7. Yun-Zi Liu, Yun-Xia Wang, Chun-Lei Jiang, "Inflammation: The Common Pathway of Stress-Related Diseases," *Frontiers Human Neuroscience* 11 (2017): 316, https://doi.org/10.3389/fnhum.2017.00316.
8. Marta Tristan Asensi, Antonia Napoletano, Franceesco Sofi, and Monica Dinu, "Low-Grade Inflammation and Ultra-Processed Foods Consumption: A Review," *Nutrients* 15, no. 6 (2023): 1546, https://doi.org/10.3390/nu15061546.
9. Patricia González, Pedro Lozano, Gaspar Ros, Francisco Solano, "Hyperglycemia and Oxidative Stress: An Integral, Updated and Critical Overview of Their Metabolic Interconnections," *International Journal of Molecular Sciences* 24, no. 11 (2023): 9352, https://doi.org/10.3390/ijms24119352.
10. Zahraa Al Bander, Marloes Dekker Nitert, Aya Mousa, and Negar Naderpoor, "The Gut Microbiota and Inflammation: An Overview," *International Journal of Environmental Research and Public Health* 17, no. 20 (2020): 7618, https://doi.org/10.3390/ijerph17207618.
11. Deepesh Khanna, Siya Khanna, Pragya Khanna, Payal Kahar, and Bhavesh M. Patel, "Obesity: A Chronic Low-Grade Inflammation and Its Markers," *Cureus* 14, no. 2 (2022): e22711, https://doi.org/10.7759/cureus.22711.
12. Janet M. Mullington, Norah S. Simpson, Hans K. Meier-Ewert, and Monika Haack, "Sleep Loss and Inflammation," *Best Practice & Research Clinical Endocrinology & Metabolism* 24, no. 5 (2010): 775–84, https://doi.org/10.1016/j.beem.2010.08.014.
13. Patricia A. Thompson, Mahin Khatami, Carolyn J. Baglole, Jun Sun, Shelley A. Harris, Eun-Yi Moon et al., "Environmental Immune Disruptors, Inflammation and Cancer Risk," *Carcinogenesis* 36, Suppl 1 (2015): S232–53, https://doi.org/10.1093/carcin/bgv038.
14. Kenneth J. Mukamal, "The Effects of Smoking and Drinking on Cardiovascular Disease and Risk Factors," *Alcohol Research and Health* 29, no. 3 (2006): 199–202.

How the Cortisol Reset Plan Will Help You Thrive

1. Sara Gottfried, *The Hormone Cure: Reclaim Balance, Sleep, Sex Drive, and Vitality Naturally with the Gottfried Protocol* (Scribner, 2013): 24–26.
2. Charles Duhigg, *The Power of Habit: Why We Do What We Do in Life and Business* (Random House, 2012): 4–30.

3. Norman Rosenthal, "Habit Formation," *Psychology Today*, accessed November 30, 2011.
4. James Clearn, "How to Build New Habits by Taking Advantage of Old Ones," accessed May 13, 2025, https://jamesclear.com/habit-stacking; Tiny Habits, accessed May 13, 2025, https://tinyhabits.com/.

Step One: Eat a Nutrient-Dense Diet

1. Zev Schuman-Olivier, Marcelo Trombka, David A. Lovas, Judson A. Brewer, David R. Vago, Richa Gawande et al., "Mindfulness and Behavior Change," *Harvard Review of Psychiatry* 28, no. 6 (2020): 371–94, https://doi.org/10.1097/HRP.0000000000000277.
2. Abraham Tobias and Nazia M. Sadiq, *Physiology, Gastrointestinal Nervous Control,* (StatPearls, 2002).
3. Mauro Finicelli, Anna Di Salle, Umberto Galderisi, and Gianfranco Peluso, "The Mediterranean Diet: An Update of the Clinical Trials," *Nutrients* 14, no. 14 (2022): 2956, https://doi.org/10.3390/nu14142956.
4. US Department of Agriculture and US Department of Health and Human Services, *Dietary Guidelines for Americans, 2020–2025*, 9th edition, updated December 2020, https://www.dietaryguidelines.gov/sites/default/files/2020-12/Dietary_Guidelines_for_Americans_2020-2025.pdf.
5. John W. Carbone and Stefan M. Pasiakos, "Dietary Protein and Muscle Mass: Translating Science to Application and Health Benefit," *Nutrients* 11, no. 5 (2019): 1136, https://doi.org/10.3390/nu11051136; Stuart M. Phillips, Stephanie Chevalier, and Heather J. Leidy, "Protein 'Requirements' Beyond the RDA: Implications for Optimizing Health," *Applied Physiology, Nutrition, and Metabolism* 41, no. 5 (2016): 565–72, https://doi.org/10.1139/apnm-2015-0550; Everson A. Nunes, Lauren Colenso-Semple, Sean R. McKellar, Thomas Yau, Muhammad Usman Ali, Donna Fitzpatrick-Lewis, et al., "Systematic Review and Meta-Analysis of Protein Intake to Support Muscle Mass and Function in Healthy Adults," *Journal of Cachexia Sarcopenia Muscle* 13, no. 2 (2022): 795–810, https://doi.org/10.1002/jcsm.12922.
6. Yasuda Jun, Tomita Toshiki, Arimitsu Takuma, and Fujita Satoshi, "Evenly Distributed Protein Intake Over 3 Meals Augments Resistance Exercise-Induced Muscle Hypertrophy in Healthy Young Men," *Journal of Nutrition* 150, no. 7 (2020): 1845–51, https://doi.org/10.1093/jn/nxaa101.
7. "Food Data Central," US Department of Agriculture, accessed June 5, 2025, https://fdc.nal.usda.gov/.

8. "Carbohydrates," Health Direct, accessed June 5, 2025, https://www.healthdirect.gov.au/carbohydrates.
9. "Fats and Cholesterol," The Nutrition Source, Harvard T. H. Chan School of Public Health, accessed June 5, 2025, https://nutritionsource.hsph.harvard.edu/what-should-you-eat/fats-and-cholesterol/.
10. Consuelo Santa-María, Soledad López-Enríquez, Sergio Montserrat-de la Paz, Isabel Geniz, María Edith Reyes-Quiroz, Manuela Moreno, et al., "Update on Anti-Inflammatory Molecular Mechanisms Induced by Oleic Acid," *Nutrients* 15, no. 1 (2023): 224, https://doi.org/10.3390/nu15010224.
11. Lee Hooper, Nicole Martin, Oluseyi F Jimoh, Christian Kirk, Eve Foster, and Asmaa S Abdelhamid, "Reduction in Saturated Fat Intake for Cardiovascular Disease," *Cochrane Database of Systematic Reviews* 8 (2020): CD011737, https://doi.org/10.1002/14651858.CD011737.pub3.
12. Riya Ganguly and Grant N. Pierce, "Trans Fat Involvement in Cardiovascular Disease," *Molecular Nutrition & Food Research* 56, no. 7 (2012): 1090–96, https://doi.org/10.1002/mnfr.201100700.
13. Danielle Swanson, Robert Block, and Shaker A. Mousa, "Omega-3 Fatty Acids EPA and DHA: Health Benefits Throughout Life," *Advances in Nutrition* 3, no. 1 (2012): 1–7, https://doi.org/10.3945/an.111.000893.
14. Mark L. Dreher, Feon W. Cheng, and Nikki A. Ford, "A Comprehensive Review of Hass Avocado Clinical Trials, Observational Studies, and Biological Mechanisms," *Nutrients* 13, no. 12 (2021): 4376, https://doi.org/10.3390/nu13124376.
15. James J. DiNicolantonio and James H. O'Keefe, "Importance of Maintaining a Low Omega-6/Omega-3 Ratio for Reducing Inflammation," *Open Heart* 5, no. 2 (2018): e000946, https://doi.org/10.1136/openhrt-2018–000946.
16. Maryam S. Farvid, Elkhansa Sidahmed, Nicholas D. Spence, Kingsly Mante Angua, Bernard A. Rosner, and Junaidah B. Barnett, "Consumption of Red Meat and Processed Meat and Cancer Incidence: A Systematic Review and Meta-Analysis of Prospective Studies," *European Journal of Epidemiology* 36, no. 9 (2021): 937–51, https://doi.org/10.1007/s10654–021–00741–9.
17. "IARC Monographs Evaluate Red and Processed Meats," World Health Organization, published October 26, 2015, https://www.emro.who.int/noncommunicable-diseases/highlights/red-and-processed-meats-cause-cancer.html.
18. Marta Tristan Asensi, Antonia Napoletano, Francesco Sofi, and Monica Dinu, "Low-Grade Inflammation and Ultra-Processed Foods Consumption: A Review," *Nutrients* 15, no. 6 (2023): 1546, https://doi.org/10.3390/nu15061546.

19. US Food and Drug Administration, "Trans Fat," accessed 7/29/2025, https://www.fda.gov/food/food-additives-petitions/trans-fat.
20. Jotham Suez, Tal Korem, Gili Zilberman-Schapira, Eran Segal, and Eran Elinav, "Non-Caloric Artificial Sweeteners and the Microbiome: Findings and Challenges," *Gut Microbes* 6, no. 2 (2015): 149–55, https://doi.org/10.1080/19490976.2015.1017700.
21. Andrea Conz, Mario Salmona, and Luisa Diomede, "Effect of Non-Nutritive Sweeteners on the Gut Microbiota," *Nutrients* 15, no. 8 (2023): 1869, https://doi.org/10.3390/nu15081869.
22. Andreia Oliveira, Fernando Rodríguez-Artalejo, and Carla Lopes, "Alcohol Intake and Systemic Markers of Inflammation—Shape of the Association According to Sex and Body Mass Index," *Alcohol and Alcoholism* 45, no. 2 (2010): 119–25, https://doi.org/10.1093/alcalc/agp092.
23. Eugenia Lauret and Luis Rodrigo, "Celiac Disease and Autoimmune-Associated Conditions," *BioMed Research International* 2013, no. 1 (2013): 127589, https://doi.org/10.1155/2013/127589.
24. Rosa Krajmalnik-Brown, Zehra-Esra Ilhan, Dae-Wook Kang, and John K. DiBaise, "Effects of Gut Microbes on Nutrient Absorption and Energy Regulation," *Nutrition in Clinical Practice* 27, no. 2 (2012): 201–14, https://doi.org/10.1177/0884533611436116.
25. Michelle G. Rooks and Wendy S. Garrett, "Gut microbiota, Metabolites, and Host Immunity," *Nature Reviews Immunology* 16, no. 6 (2016): 341–52, https://doi.org/10.1038/nri.2016.42.
26. Elaine Patterson, Paul M. Ryan, John F. Cryan, Timothy G. Dinan, R. Paul Ross, Gerald F. Fitzgerald, and Catherine Stanton, "Gut Microbiota, Obesity and Diabetes," *Postgraduate Medical Journal* 92, no. 1087 (2016): 286–300, https://doi.org/10.1136/postgradmedj-2015-133285.
27. John F. Cryan and Timothy G. Dinan, "Mind-Altering Microorganisms: The Impact of the Gut Microbiota on Brain and Behaviour," *Nature Reviews Neuroscience* 13, no. 10 (2012): 701–12, https://doi.org/10.1038/nrn3346.
28. H. X. Chong, N. A. A. Yusoff, Y.-Y. Hor, L.-C. Lew, M. H. Jaafar, S.-B. Choi at al., "*Lactobacillus plantarum* DR7 Alleviates Stress and Anxiety in Adults: A Randomised, Double-Blind, Placebo-Controlled Study," *Beneficial Microbes* 10, no. 4 (2019): 355–73, https://doi.org/10.3920/BM2018.0135.
29. Jing Ji, Weilin Jin, Shuang-Jiang Liu, Zuoyi Jiao, and Xiangkai Li, "Probiotics, Prebiotics, and Postbiotics in Health and Disease," *MedComm* 4, no. 6 (2023): e420, https://doi.org/10.1002/mco2.420.

30. Janine A. Higgins, "Resistant Starch: Metabolic Effects and Potential Health Benefits," *Journal of AOAC International* 87, no. 3 (2019): 761–68. https://doi.org/10.1093/jaoac/87.3.761.
31. Xiaofei Wang, Yue Qi, and Hao Zheng, "Dietary Polyphenol, Gut Microbiota, and Health Benefits," *Antioxidants* 11, no. 6 (2022): 1212, https://doi.org/10.3390/antiox11061212.
32. A. P. Allen, W. Hutch, Y. E. Borre, P. J. Kennedy, A. Temko, G. Boylan et al., "*Bifidobacterium longum* 1714 as a Translational Psychobiotic: Modulation of Stress, Electrophysiology and Neurocognition in Healthy Volunteers," *Translational Psychiatry* 6, no. 11 (2016): e93, https://doi .org/10.1038/tp.2016.191; J. Wang, C. Braun, E. F. Murphy and P. Enck, "Bifidobacterium longum 1714™ Strain Modulates Brain Activity of Healthy Volunteers During Social Stress," *American Journal of Gastroenterology* 114, no. 7 (2019): 1152–62.
33. Huiying Wang, Christoph Braun, Eileen F Murphy, and Paul Enck, "*Bifidobacterium longum* 1714™ Strain Modulates Brain Activity of Healthy Volunteers During Social Stress," *American Journal of Gastroenterology* 114, no. 7 (2019): 1152–62, https://doi.org/10.14309 /ajg.0000000000000203.
34. A. C. Rodrigues, D. C. Cara, S. H. Fretez, F. Q. Cunha, E. C. Vieira, J. R. Nicoli, and L. Q. Vieira, "*Saccharomyces boulardii* Stimulates sIgA Production and the Phagocytic System of Gnotobiotic Mice," *Journal of Applied Microbiology* 89, no. 3 (2000): 404–14, https://doi.org/10.1046 /j.1365-2672.2000.01128.x.
35. I. J. de Oliveira, V. V. de Souza, V. Motta, and S. L. Da-Silva, "Effects of Oral Vitamin C Supplementation on Anxiety in Students: A Double-Blind, Randomized, Placebo-Controlled Trial," *Pakistan Journal of Biological Sciences* 18, no. 1 (2015): 11–18, https://doi.org/10.3923/pjbs .2015.11.18.
36. N. B. Boyle, C. Lawton, and L. Dye, "The Effects of Magnesium Supplementation on Subjective Anxiety and Stress—A Systematic Review," *Nutrients* 9, no. 5 (2017): 429, https://doi.org/10.3390 /nu9050429.
37. G. Pickering, A. Mazur, M. Trousselard, P. Bienkowski, N. Yaltsewa, M. Amessou, L. Noah, and E. Pouteau, "Magnesium Status and Stress: The Vicious Circle Concept Revisited," *Nutrients* 12, no. 12 (2020): 3672, https://doi.org/10.3390/nu12123672.
38. K. Kostov, "Effects of Magnesium Deficiency on Mechanisms of Insulin Resistance in Type 2 Diabetes: Focusing on the Processes of Insulin Secretion and Signaling," *International Journal of Molecular Sciences* 20, no. 6 (2019): 1351, https://doi.org/10.3390/ijms20061351.

39. National Institutes of Health, Office of Dietary Supplements, "Magnesium: Fact Sheet for Health Professionals," updated June 2, 2022, https://ods.od.nih.gov/factsheets/Magnesium-HealthProfessional/.
40. Y. Osher and R. H. Belmaker, "Omega-3 Fatty Acids in Depression: A Review of Three Studies," *CNS Neuroscience & Therapeutics* 15, no. 2 (2009): 128–33, https://doi.org/10.1111/j.1755-5949.2008.00061.x.
41. US Department of Agriculture and US Department of Health and Human Services, *Dietary Guidelines for Americans, 2020–2025*, 9th ed., updated December 2020, https://www.dietaryguidelines.gov/sites/default/files/2020-12/Dietary_Guidelines_for_Americans_2020-2025.pdf.
42. David O. Kennedy, "B Vitamins and the Brain: Mechanisms, Dose and Efficacy—A Review," *Nutrients* 8, no. 2 (2016): 68, https://doi.org/10.3390/nu8020068.
43. A. Tarasov Iu, V. M. Sheibak, and A. G. Moiseenok, "Adrenal Cortex Functional Activity in Pantothenate Deficiency and the Administration of the Vitamin or Its Derivatives," *Voprosy Pitaniia* 4 (1985): 51–54.

Step Two: Balance Your Blood Sugar

1. Joan Araújo, Jianwen Cai, and June Stevens, "Prevalence of Optimal Metabolic Health in American Adults: National Health and Nutrition Examination Survey 2009–2016," *Metabolic Syndrome and Related Disorders* 17, no. 1 (2019): 46–52, https://doi.org/10.1089/met.2018.0105.
2. N. W. S. Chew, C. H. Ng, D. J. H. Tan, G. Kong, C. Lin, Y. H. Chin, et al., "The Global Burden of Metabolic Disease: Data from 2000 to 2019." *Cell Metabolism* 35, no. 3 (2023): 414–428.e3, https://doi.org/10.1016/j.cmet.2023.02.003.
3. "Blood Glucose and A1C: Understanding Diabetes Diagnosis," American Diabetes Association, accessed June 5, 2025, https://diabetes.org/about-diabetes/diagnosis.
4. A. Ceriello and S. Colagiuri, "International Diabetes Federation Guideline for Management of Postmeal Glucose: a Review of Recommendations," *Diabetic Medicine* 25, no. 10 (2008): 1151–56, https://doi.org/10.1111/j.1464-5491.2008.02565.x.
5. Hye Seung Jung, "Clinical Implications of Glucose Variability: Chronic Complications of Diabetes," *Endocrinology and Metabolism (Seoul)* 30, no. 2 (2015): 167–74, https://doi.org/10.3803/EnM.2015.30.2.167.
6. S. Penckofer, L. Quinn, M. Byrn, C. Ferrans, M. Miller, and P. Strange, "Does Glycemic Variability Impact Mood and Quality of Life?,"

Diabetes Technology & Therapeutics 14, no. 4 (2012): 303–10, https://doi.org/10.1089/dia.2011.0191; K. T. Watson, J. F. Simard, V. W. Henderson, L. Nutkiewicz, F. Lamers, C. Nasca et al., "Incident Major Depressive Disorder Predicted by Three Measures of Insulin Resistance: A Dutch Cohort Study," *American Journal of Psychiatry* 178, no. 10 (2021): 914–20, https://doi.org/10.1176/appi.ajp.2021.20101479; Lorenzo Del Moro, Eugenia Rota, Elenamaria Pirovano, and Innocenzo Rainero, "Migraine, Brain Glucose Metabolism and the 'Neuroenergetic' Hypothesis: A Scoping Review," *Journal of Pain* 23, no. 8 (2022): 1294–1317, https://doi.org/10.1016/j.jpain.2022.02.006; I. D. Iyegha, A. Y. Chieh, B. M. Bryant, and L. Li, "Associations Between Poor Sleep and Glucose Intolerance in Prediabetes," *Psychoneuroendocrinology* 110 (2019): 104444, https://doi.org/10.1016/j.psyneuen.2019.104444; Nathalie de Rekeneire, Rita Peila, Jingzhong Ding, Lisa H. Colbert, Marjolein Visser, Ronald I. Shorr et al., "Diabetes, Hyperglycemia, and Inflammation in Older Individuals: The Health, Aging and Body Composition Study," *Diabetes Care* 29, no. 8 (2006): 1902–08, https://doi.org/10.2337/dc05-2327; Andrew M. Freeman, Luis A. Acevedo, and Nicholas Pennings, *StatPearls* (StatPearls, 2025), https://www.ncbi.nlm.nih.gov/books/NBK507839/; Abigail Dove, Jiao Wang, Huijie Huang, Michelle M. Dunk, Sakura Sakakibara, Marc Guitart-Masip et al., "Diabetes, Prediabetes, and Brain Aging: The Role of Healthy Lifestyle," *Diabetes Care* 47 , no. 10 (2024): 1794–1802, https://doi.org/10.2337/dc24-0860.

7. Diana Gentilcore, Reawika Chaikomin, Karen L. Jones, Antonietta Russo, Christine Feinle-Bisset, Judith M. Wishart, et al., "Effects of Fat on Gastric Emptying of and the Glycemic, Insulin, and Incretin Responses to a Carbohydrate Meal in Type 2 Diabetes," *Journal of Clinical Endocrinology & Metabolism* 91, no. 6 (2006): 2062–67, https://doi.org/10.1210/jc.2005-2644.
8. J. Ma, J. E. Stevens, K. Cukier, A. F. Maddox, J. M. Wishart, K. L. Jones et al., "Effects of a Protein Preload on Gastric Emptying, Glycemia, and Gut Hormones after a Carbohydrate Meal in Diet-Controlled Type 2 Diabetes," *Diabetes Care* 32, no. 9 (2009): 1600–2, https://doi.org/10.2337/dc09-0723.
9. A. Reynolds, J. Mann, J. Cummings, N. Winter, E. Mete, and L. Te Morenga, "Carbohydrate Quality and Human Health: A Series of Systematic Reviews and Meta-Analyses," *Lancet* 393, no. 10170 (2019): 434–45, https://doi.org/10.1016/S0140-6736(18)31809-9.
10. US Department of Agriculture and US Department of Health and Human Services, *Dietary Guidelines for Americans, 2020–2025*, 9th ed.,

updated December 2020, https://www.dietaryguidelines.gov/sites/default/files/2020-12/Dietary_Guidelines_for_Americans_2020-2025.pdf.

11. "Rough Up Your Diet: Fit More Fiber into Your Day," *NIH*: News in Health, accessed 7/29/2025, https://newsinhealth.nih.gov/2019/07/rough-up-your-diet.
12. A. N. Reynolds, A. P. Akerman, and J. Mann, "Dietary Fibre and Whole Grains in Diabetes Management: Systematic Review and Meta-Analyses," *PLoS Medicine* 17, no. 3 (2020): e1003053, https://doi.org/10.1371/journal.pmed.1003053.
13. M. O. Weickert and A. F. H. Pfeiffer, "Impact of Dietary Fiber Consumption on Insulin Resistance and the Prevention of Type 2 Diabetes." *Journal of Nutrition* 148, no. 1 (2018): 7–12, https://doi.org/10.1093/jn/nxx008. PMID: 29378044.
14. M. C. W. Myhrstad, H. Tunsjø, C. Charnock, and V. H. Telle-Hansen, "Dietary Fiber, Gut Microbiota, and Metabolic Regulation-Current Status in Human Randomized Trials," *Nutrients* 12, no. 3 (2020): 859, https://doi.org/10.3390/nu12030859.
15. J. Ji, W. Jin, S. J. Liu, Z. Jiao, X. Li, "Probiotics, Prebiotics, and Postbiotics in Health and Disease," *MedComm* 4, no. 6 (2023): e420, https://doi.org/10.1002/mco2.420.
16. J. A. Gwin and H. J. Leidy, "A Review of the Evidence Surrounding the Effects of Breakfast Consumption on Mechanisms of Weight Management," *Advances in Nutrition* 9, no. 6 (2018): 717–25, https://doi.org/10.1093/advances/nmy047.
17. D. Jakubowicz, J. Wainstein, Z. Landau, I. Raz, B. Ahren, N. Chapnik, et al., "Influences of Breakfast on Clock Gene Expression and Postprandial Glycemia in Healthy Individuals and Individuals With Diabetes: A Randomized Clinical Trial," *Diabetes Care* 40, no. 11 (2017): 1573–79, https://doi.org/10.2337/dc16-2753.
18. B. L. Reddy, V. S. Reddy, M. J. Saier Jr,. "Health Benefits of Intermittent Fasting," *Microbial Physiology* 34, no. 1 (2024): 142–52, https://doi.org/10.1159/000540068.
19. D. Jakubowicz, M. Barnea M, J. Wainstein, and O. Froy, "High Caloric Intake at Breakfast Vs. Dinner Differentially Influences Weight Loss of Overweight and Obese Women," *Obesity (Silver Spring)* 21, no. 12 (2013): 2504–12, https://doi.org/10.1002/oby.20460.
20. L. O. Pereira and A. H. Lancha, "Effect of Insulin and Contraction up on Glucose Transport in Skeletal Muscle," *Progress in Biophysics &Molecular Biology* 84, no. 1 (2004): 1–27, https://doi.org/10.1016/s0079-6107(03)00055-5.

21. A. J. Buffey, M. P. Herring, C. K. Langley, A. E. Donnelly, and B. P. Carson, "The Acute Effects of Interrupting Prolonged Sitting Time in Adults with Standing and Light-Intensity Walking on Biomarkers of Cardiometabolic Health in Adults: a Systematic Review and Meta-Analysis," *Sports Medicine* 52, no. 8 (2022): 1765–87, https://doi.org/10.1007/s40279-022-01649-4.
22. A. N. Reynolds, J. L. Mann, S. Williams, and B. J. Venn, "Advice to Walk after Meals Is More Effective for Lowering Postprandial Glycaemia in Type 2 Diabetes Mellitus than Advice That Does Not Specify Timing: A Randomised Crossover Study," *Diabetologia* 59, no. 12 (2016): 2572–78, https://doi.org/10.1007/s00125-016-4085-2.
23. A. Caplin, F. S. Chen, M. R. Beauchamp, and E. Puterman, "The Effects of Exercise Intensity on the Cortisol Response to a Subsequent Acute Psychosocial Stressor," *Psychoneuroendocrinology* 131 (2021): 105336, https://doi.org/10.1016/j.psyneuen.2021.105336.
24. N. Veronese, L. J. Dominguez, D. Pizzol, J. Demurtas, L. Smith, and M. Barbagallo. "Oral Magnesium Supplementation for Treating Glucose Metabolism Parameters in People with or at Risk of Diabetes: A Systematic Review and Meta-Analysis of Double-Blind Randomized Controlled Trials," *Nutrients* 13, no. 11 (2021): 4074, https://doi.org/10.3390/nu13114074.
25. P. J. Havel, "A Scientific Review: the Role of Chromium in Insulin Resistance," *Diabetes Education* Supplement (2024): 2–14, https://pubmed.ncbi.nlm.nih.gov/15208835/.
26. N. Mohd Ghozali, N. Giribabu, and N. Salleh, "Mechanisms Linking Vitamin D Deficiency to Impaired Metabolism: An Overview," *International Journal of Endocrinology* 2022 (2022): 6453882, https://doi.org/10.1155/2022/6453882.
27. M. Akbari, V. Ostadmohammadi, K. B. Lankarani, R. Tabrizi, F. Kolahdooz, S. R. Khatibi, and Z. Asemi, "The Effects of Alpha-Lipoic Acid Supplementation on Glucose Control and Lipid Profiles among Patients with Metabolic Diseases: A Systematic Review and Meta-Analysis of Randomized Controlled Trials," *Metabolism* 87 (2018): 56–69, https://doi.org/10.1016/j.metabol.2018.07.002.
28. B. Kalra, S. Kalra, and J. B. Sharma, "The Inositols and Polycystic Ovary Syndrome," *Indian Journal of Endocrinology and Metabolism* 20, no. 5 (2016): 720–24, https://doi.org/10.4103/2230-8210.189231.
29. M. Hajimonfarednejad, M. Nimrouzi, M. Heydari, M. M. Zarshenas, M. J. Raee, and B. N. Jahromi, "Insulin Resistance Improvement by Cinnamon Powder in Polycystic Ovary Syndrome: A Randomized

Double-Blind Placebo Controlled Clinical Trial" *Phytotherapy Research* 32, no. 2 (2018): 276–83, https://doi.org/10.1002/ptr.5970.

30. Richard A. Anderson, Zhiwei Zhan, Rencai Luo, Xiuhua Guo, Qingqing Guo, Jin Zhou, Jiang Kong, Paul A. Davis, and Barbara J. Stoecker, "Cinnamon Extract Lowers Glucose, Insulin and Cholesterol in People with Elevated Serum Glucose," *Journal of Traditional and Complementary Medicine* 6, no. 4 (2016): 332–36.
31. K. Hanhineva, R. Törrönen, I. Bondia-Pons, J. Pekkinen, M. Kolehmainen, H. Mykkänen, and K. Poutanen, "Impact of Dietary Polyphenols on Carbohydrate Metabolism," *International Journal of Molecular Sciences* 11, no. 4 (2010):1365–402, https://doi.org/10.3390/ijms11041365.
32. Y. Kim, J. B. Keogh, and P. M. Clifton, "Polyphenols and Glycemic Control," *Nutrients* 8, no. 1 (2016): 17, https://doi.org/10.3390/nu8010017.

Step Three: Regulate Your Circadian Rhythm

1. A. Lopez-Santamarina, A. D. C. Mondragon, A. Cardelle-Cobas, E. M. Santos, J. J. Porto-Arias, A. Cepeda, and J. M. Miranda, "Effects of Unconventional Work and Shift Work on the Human Gut Microbiota and the Potential of Probiotics to Restore Dysbiosis," *Nutrients* 15, no. 3 (2023): 3070, https://doi.org/10.3390/nu15133070; H. Mortaş, S. Bilici, and T. Karakan, "The Circadian Disruption of Night Work Alters Gut Microbiota Consistent with Elevated Risk for Future Metabolic and Gastrointestinal Pathology," *Chronobiology International* 37, no. 7 (2020): 1067–81, https://doi.org/10.1080/07420528.2020.1778717; Q. Liu, J. Shi, P. Duan, B. Liu, T. Li, C. Wang, H. Li, T. Yang, Y. Gan, X. Wang, S. Cao, and Z. Lu, "Is Shift Work Associated with a Higher Risk of Overweight or Obesity? a Systematic Review of Observational Studies with Meta-Analysis," *International Journal of Epidemiology* 47, no. 6 (2018): 1956–71, https://doi.org/10.1093/ije/dyy079; C. Vetter, H. S. Dashti, J. M. Lane, S. G. Anderson, E. S. Schernhammer, M. K. Rutter, R. Saxena, F. A. J. L. Scheer, "Night Shift Work, Genetic Risk, and Type 2 Diabetes in the UK Biobank," *Diabetes Care* 41, no. 4 (2018): 762–69, https://doi.org/10.2337/dc17–1933; D. L. Brown, D. Feskanich, B. N. Sánchez, K. M. Rexrode, E. S. Schernhammer, and L. D. Lisabeth, "Rotating Night Shift Work and the Risk of Ischemic Stroke," *American Journal of Epidemiology* 169, no. 11(2009): 1370–77, https://doi.org/10.1093/aje/kwp056.
2. J. A. Mohawk, C. B. Green, and J. S. Takahashi, "Central and Peripheral Circadian Clocks in Mammals," *Annual Review of Neuroscience* 35

(2012): 445–62, https://doi.org/10.1146/annurev-neuro-060909-153128.

3. B. S. McEwen and I. N. Karatsoreos, "Sleep Deprivation and Circadian Disruption: Stress, Allostasis, and Allostatic Load," *Sleep Medicine Clinics* 10, no. 1 (2015): 1–10, https://doi.org/10.1016/j.jsmc.2014.11.007.
4. M. I. Silvani, R. Werder, and C. Perret, "The Influence of Blue Light on Sleep, Performance and Wellbeing in Young Adults: A Systematic Review," *Frontiers in Physiology* 13 (2022): 943108, https://doi.org/10.3389/fphys.2022.943108.
5. R. Leproult, E. F. Colecchia, M. L'Hermite-Balériaux, and E. Van Cauter, "Transition from Dim to Bright Light in the Morning Induces an Immediate Elevation of Cortisol Levels," *Journal of Clinical Endocrinology and Metabolism* 86, no. 1 (2001): 151–57, https://doi.org/10.1210/jcem.86.1.7102.
6. A. van Maanen, A. M. Meijer, K. B. van der Heijden, and F. J. Oort, "The Effects of Light Therapy on Sleep Problems: A Systematic Review and Meta-Analysis," *Sleep Medicine Reviews* 29 (2016): 52–62, https://doi.org/10.1016/j.smrv.2015.08.009.
7. F. Damiola, N. Le Minh, N. Preitner, B. Kornmann, F. Fleury-Olela, and U. Schibler, "Restricted Feeding Uncouples Circadian Oscillators in Peripheral Tissues from the Central Pacemaker in the Suprachiasmatic Nucleus," *Genes & Development* 14, no. 23 (2000): 2950–61, https://doi.org/10.1101/gad.183500. PMID: 11114885.
8. J. K. Srivastava, E. Shankar, and S. Gupta, "Chamomile: A Herbal Medicine of the Past with Bright Future," *Molecular Medicine Reports* 3, no. 6 (2010): 895–901, https://doi.org/10.3892/mmr.2010.377; S. M. Chang and C. H. Chen, "Effects of an Intervention with Drinking Chamomile Tea on Sleep Quality and Depression in Sleep Disturbed Postnatal Women: A Randomized Controlled Trial," *Journal of Advanced Nursing* 72, no. 2 (2016): 306–15, https://doi.org/10.1111/jan.12836.
9. J. Ghazizadeh, S. Sadigh-Eteghad, W. Marx, A. Fakhari, S. Hamedeyazdan, M. Torbati, S. Taheri-Tarighi, M. Araj-Khodaei, and M. Mirghafourvand, "The Effects of Lemon Balm (*Melissa officinalis L.*) on Depression and Anxiety in Clinical Trials: A Systematic Review and Meta-Analysis," *Phytotherapy Research* 35, no. 12 (2021): 6690–705, https://doi.org/10.1002/ptr.7252.
10. S. M. Elsas, D. J. Rossi, J. Raber, G. White, C. A. Seeley, W. L. Gregory, C. Mohr, T. Pfankuch, and A. Soumyanath, "*Passiflora incarnata L.* (passionflower) Extracts Elicit GABA Currents in Hippocampal

Neurons in Vitro, and Show Anxiogenic and Anticonvulsant Effects in Vivo, Varying with Extraction Method," *Phytomedicine* 17, no. 12 (2010): 940–49, https://doi.org/10.1016/j.phymed.2010.03.002.

11. B. M. Gabriel and J. R. Zierath, "Circadian Rhythms and Exercise: Re-Setting the Clock in Metabolic Disease," *Nature Reviews Endocrinology* 15, no. 4 (2019): 197–206, https://doi.org/10.1038/s41574-018-0150-x.
12. H. Chtourou and N. Souissi, "The Effect of Training at a Specific Time of Day: A Review," *Journal of Strength and Conditioning Research* 26, no. 7 (2012): 1984–2005, https://doi.org/10.1519/JSC.0b013e31825770a7.
13. J. Stutz, R. Eiholzer, and C. M. Spengler, "Effects of Evening Exercise on Sleep in Healthy Participants: A Systematic Review and Meta-Analysis," *Sports Medicine* 49, no. 2 (2019): 269–87, https://doi.org/10.1007/s40279-018-1015-0.
14. B. S. McEwen and I. N. Karatsoreos, "Sleep Deprivation and Circadian Disruption: Stress, Allostasis, and Allostatic Load," *Sleep Medicine Clinics* 10, no. 1 (2015): 1–10, https://doi.org/10.1016/j.jsmc.2014.11.007.
15. K. Kräuchi, C. Cajochen, E. Werth, and A. Wirz-Justice, "Functional Link between Distal Vasodilation and Sleep-Onset Latency?," *American Journal of Physiology-Regulatory, Integrative, and Comparative Physiology* 278, no. 3 (2000): R741–8, https://doi.org/10.1152/ajpregu.2000.278.3.R741.

Step Four: Exercise for Mind and Body Health

1. "Benefits of Physical Activity," Centers for Disease Control and Prevention, published April 24, 2024, https://www.cdc.gov/physical-activity-basics/benefits/index.html.
2. Marni N. Silverman and Patricia A. Deuster, "Biological Mechanisms Underlying the Role of Physical Fitness in Health and Resilience," *Interface Focus* 4, no. 5 (2014): 20140040, https://doi.org/ 10.1098/rsfs.2014.0040.
3. M. Nowacka-Chmielewska, K. Grabowska, M. Grabowski, P. Meybohm, M. Burek, and A. Małecki, "Running from Stress: Neurobiological Mechanisms of Exercise-Induced Stress Resilience," *International Journal of Molecular Sciences* 23, no. 21 (2022): 13348, https://doi.org/10.3390/ijms232113348.
4. N. Skoluda, L. Dettenborn, T. Stalder, C. Kirschbaum, "Elevated Hair Cortisol Concentrations in Endurance Athletes," *Psychoneuroendocrinology* 37, no. 5 (2012): 611–17, https://doi.org/10.1016/j.psyneuen.2011.09.001.

5. US Department of Health and Human Services, *Physical Activity Guidelines for Americans*, 2nd ed. published 2018, https://health.gov/sites/default/files/2019-09/Physical_Activity_Guidelines_2nd_edition.pdf.
6. P. Kokkinos, C. Faselis, I. B. H. Samuel, A. Pittaras, M. Doumas, R. Murphy, M. S. Heimall, X. Sui, J. Zhang, and J. Myers, "Cardiorespiratory Fitness and Mortality Risk across the Spectra of Age, Race, and Sex," *Journal of the American College of Cardiology* 80, no. 6 (2022): 598–609, https://doi.org/10.1016/j.jacc.2022.05.031.
7. S. F. Sleiman, J. Henry, R. Al-Haddad, L. El Hayek, E. Abou Haidar, T. Stringer, D. Ulja, S. S. Karuppagounder, E. B. Holson, R. R. Ratan, I. Ninan, and M. V. Chao, "Exercise Promotes the Expression of Brain Derived Neurotrophic Factor (BDNF) Through the Action of the Ketone Body β-hydroxybutyrate," *Elife* 5 (2016): e15092, https://doi.org/10.7554/eLife.15092.
8. I. D. Morres, A. Hatzigeorgiadis, A. Stathi, N. Comoutos, C. Arpin-Cribbie, C. Krommidas, and Y. Theodorakis, "Aerobic Exercise for Adult Patients with Major Depressive Disorder in Mental Health Services: A Systematic Review and Meta-Analysis," *Depression and Anxiety* 36, no. 1 (2019): 39–53, https://doi.org/10.1002/da.22842.
9. D. E. Warburton, C. W. Nicol, and S. S. Bredin, "Health Benefits of Physical Activity: The Evidence," *Canadian Medical Association Journal* 174, no. 6 (2006): 801–9, https://doi.org/10.1503/cmaj.051351.
10. M. J. Niemann, L. A. Tucker, B. W. Bailey, L. E. Davidson, "Strength Training and Insulin Resistance: The Mediating Role of Body Composition," *Journal of Diabetes Research* 2020 (2020): 7694825, https://doi.org/10.1155/2020/7694825.
11. P. Srikanthan and A. S. Karlamangla, "Muscle Mass Index as a Predictor of Longevity in Older Adults," *American Journal of Medicine* 127, no. 6 (2014): 547–53, https://doi.org/10.1016/j.amjmed.2014.02.007.
12. T. W. Kim, S. H. Lee, K. H. Choi, D. H. Kim, and T. K. Han, "Comparison of The Effects of Acute Exercise after Overnight Fasting and Breakfast on Energy Substrate and Hormone Levels in Obese Men," *Journal of Physical Therapy Science* 27, no. 6 (2015): 1929–32, https://doi.org/10.1589/jpts.27.1929.
13. N. Romero-Parra, R. Cupeiro, V. M. Alfaro-Magallanes, B. Rael, J. Á. Rubio-Arias, A. B. Peinado, and P. J. Benito, "Exercise-Induced Muscle Damage During the Menstrual Cycle: A Systematic Review and Meta-Analysis," *Journal of Strength and Conditioning Research* 35, no. 2 (2021): 549–61, https://doi.org/10.1519/JSC.0000000000003878.

14. J. T. Costello, F. Bieuzen, and C. M. Bleakley, "Where Are All the Female Participants in Sports and Exercise Medicine Research?," *European Journal of Sport Science* 14, no. 8 (2014): 847–51, https://doi.org/10.1080/17461391.2014.911354.
15. S. T. Sims and A. K. Heather, "Myths and Methodologies: Reducing Scientific Design Ambiguity in Studies Comparing Sexes and/or Menstrual Cycle Phases," *Experimental Physiology* 103, no. 10 (2018): 1309–17, https://doi.org/10.1113/EP086797.
16. S. Rocha-Rodrigues, M. Sousa, P. Lourenço Reis, C. Leão, B. Cardoso-Marinho, M. Massada, and J. Afonso, "Bidirectional Interactions between the Menstrual Cycle, Exercise Training, and Macronutrient Intake in Women: A Review," *Nutrients* 13, no. 2 (2021): 438, https://doi.org/10.3390/nu13020438.
17. "Perimenopause," HealthDirect, accessed June 5, 2025, https://www.healthdirect.gov.au/perimenopause.
18. S. J. Simpson, D. Raubenheimer, K. I. Black, and A. D. Conigrave, "Weight Gain During the Menopause Transition: Evidence for a Mechanism Dependent on Protein Leverage," *BJOG* 130, no. 1 (2023): 4–10, https://doi.org/10.1111/1471–0528.17290.
19. N. Chidi-Ogbolu and K. Baar, "Effect of Estrogen on Musculoskeletal Performance and Injury Risk," *Frontiers in Physiology* 15, no. 9 (2019): 1834, https://doi.org/10.3389/fphys.2018.01834.

Step Five: Build Psychological Resilience and Well-Being

1. A. M. C. Lange, M. M. Visser, R. H. J. Scholte, and C. Finkenauer, "Parental Conflicts and Posttraumatic Stress of Children in High-Conflict Divorce Families," *Journal of Child & Adolescent Trauma* 15, no. 3 (2021): 615–25, https://doi.org/10.1007/s40653–021–00410–9.
2. J. E. Sherin and C. B. Nemeroff, "Post-Traumatic Stress Disorder: The Neurobiological Impact of Psychological Trauma," *Dialogues in Clinical Neuroscience* 13, no. 3 (2011): 263–78, https://doi.org/10.31887/DCNS.2011.13.2/jsherin.
3. Polyvagal Institute, "What Is Polyvagal Theory?" accessed June 5, 2025, https://www.polyvagalinstitute.org/whatispolyvagaltheory.
4. D. J. Siegel, *The Developing Mind: How Relationships and the Brain Interact to Shape Who We Are*, 3rd ed. (Guilford Press, 2020).
5. Deb Dana, "The Science of Feeling Safe Enough to Fall in Love with Life," Rhythm of Regulation, accessed June 5, 2025, https://www.rhythmofregulation.com/glimmers.
6. G. W. Fincham, C. Strauss, J. Montero-Marin, and K. Cavanagh, "Effect of Breathwork on Stress and Mental Health: a Meta-Analysis of

Randomised-Controlled Trials," *Scientific Reports* 13. no. 1 (2023): 432, https://doi.org/10.1038/s41598–022–27247-y.

7. Melis Yilmaz Balban, Eric Neri, Manuela M. Kogon, Lara Weed, Bita Nouriani, Booil Jo, Gary Holl, Jamie M. Zeitzer, David Spiegel, and Andrew D. Huberman, "Brief Structured Respiration Practices Enhance Mood and Reduce Physiological Arousal," *Cell Reports Medicine* 4, no. 1 (2023): 100895, https://doi.org/10.1016/j.xcrm.2022.100895.
8. S. Chaitanya, A. Datta, B. Bhandari, and V. K. Sharma, "Effect of Resonance Breathing on Heart Rate Variability and Cognitive Functions in Young Adults: A Randomised Controlled Study," *Cureus* 14, no. 2 (2022): e22187, https://doi.org/10.7759/cureus.22187.
9. G. Trivedi, K. Sharma, B. Saboo, S. Kathirvel, A. Konat, V. Zapadia, P. J. Prajapati, U. Benani, K. Patel, and S. Shah, "Humming (Simple Bhramari Pranayama) as a Stress Buster: A Holter-Based Study to Analyze Heart Rate Variability (HRV) Parameters During Bhramari, Physical Activity, Emotional Stress, and Sleep," *Cureus* 15, no. 4 (2023): e37527, https://doi.org/10.7759/cureus.37527.
10. S. Rosenberg, *Accessing the Healing Power of the Vagus Nerve: Self-Help Exercises for Anxiety, Depression, Trauma, and Autism* (North Atlantic Books, 2017).
11. L. Zou, J. E. Sasaki, G. X. Wei, T. Huang, A. S. Yeung, O. B. Neto, K. W. Chen, and S. S. Hui, "Effects of Mind-Body Exercises (Tai Chi/Yoga) on Heart Rate Variability Parameters and Perceived Stress: A Systematic Review with Meta-Analysis of Randomized Controlled Trials," *Journal of Clinical Medicine* 7, no. 11 (2018): 404, https://doi.org/10.3390/jcm7110404.
12. M. Singer, *The Untethered Soul: The Journey Beyond Yourself* (New Harbinger Publications, 2007).
13. Richard C. Schwartz, *No Bad Parts: Healing Trauma and Restoring Wholeness with the Internal Family Systems Model* (Sounds True, 2021).
14. P. R. Pietromonaco and L. F. Barrett, "The Internal Working Models Concept: What Do We Really Know about the Self in Relation to Others?," *Review of General Psychology* 4, no. 2 (2000): 155–75.
15. C. J. Dahl, C. D. Wilson-Mendenhall, and R. J. Davidson, "The Plasticity of Well-Being: A Training-Based Framework for the Cultivation of Human Flourishing," *Proceedings of the National Academy of Sciences of the United States of America* 117, no. 51 (2020): 32197–206, https://doi.org/10.1073/pnas.2014859117 (2020).
16. Julianne Holt-Lunstad, "The Potential Public Health Relevance of Social Isolation and Loneliness: Prevalence, Epidemiology, and Risk

Factors," *Public Policy & Aging Report* 27, no. 4 (2017): 127–30, https://doi.org/10.1093/ppar/prx030.

17. Harvard Medical School, "Welcome to the Harvard Study of Adult Development (2015)," accessed June 5, 2025, http://www.adultdevelopmentstudy.org/.
18. Alex M. Wood, John Maltby, Raphael Gillett, P. Alex Linley, and Stephen Joseph, "The Role of Gratitude in the Development of Social Support, Stress, and Depression: Two Longitudinal Studies," *Journal of Research in Personality* 42, no. 4 (2008): 854–71, https://doi.org/10.1016/j.jrp.2007.11.003.
19. T. Singer and O. M. Klimecki, "Empathy and Compassion," *Current Biology* 24, no. 18 (2014): R875-R878, https://doi.org/10.1016/j.cub.2014.06.054.
20. D. A. Fryburg, "Kindness as a Stress Reduction-Health Promotion Intervention: A Review of the Psychobiology of Caring," *American Journal of Lifestyle Medicine* 16, no. 1 (2021): 89–100, https://doi.org/10.1177/1559827620988268.
21. K. D. Le Nguyen, J. Lin, S. B. Algoe, M. M. Brantley, S. L. Kim, J. Brantley, S. Salzberg, and B. K. Fredrickson, "Loving-Kindness Meditation Slows Biological Aging in Novices: Evidence from a 12-Week Randomized Controlled Trial," *Psychoneuroendocrinology* 108 (2019): 20–27, https://doi.org/10.1016/j.psyneuen.2019.05.020.
22. J. H. Fowler and N. A. Christakis, "Cooperative Behavior Cascades in Human Social Networks," *Proceedings of the National Academy of Sciences of the United States of America* 107, no. 12 (2010): 5334–38, https://doi.org/10.1073/pnas.0913149107.
23. S. Salzberg, *Lovingkindness: The Revolutionary Art of Happiness* (Shambhala, 1995).
24. G. Barragan-Jason, M. Loreau, C. de Mazancourt, M. C. Singer, and C. Parmesan, "Psychological and Physical Connections with Nature Improve Both Human Well-Being and Nature Conservation: A Systematic Review of Meta-Analyses," *Biological Conservation*, 277 (2023): 109842, https://doi.org/10.1016/j.biocon.2022.109842.
25. P. L. Hill and N. A. Turiano, "Purpose in Life as a Predictor of Mortality Across Adulthood," *Psychological Science* 25, no. 7 (2014): 1482–86, https://doi.org/10.1177/0956797614531799.
26. Angelina R. Sutin, Martina Luchetti, Yannick Stephan, Amanda A. Sesker, and Antonio Terracciano, "Purpose in Life and Stress: An Individual-Participant Meta-Analysis of 16 Samples," *Journal of Affective Disorders* 345 (2024): 378–85 https://doi.org/10.1016/j.jad.2023.10.149.

Appendix B: Ways to Reduce Your Toxin Exposure

1. National Institute of Environmental Science, "Pesticides," accessed June 5, 2025, https://www.niehs.nih.gov/health/topics/agents/pesticides.
2. Y. Wang and H. Qian, "Phthalates and Their Impacts on Human Health," *Healthcare (Basel)* 9, no. 5 (2021): 603, https://doi.org/10.3390/healthcare9050603.
3. J. Lincho, R. C. Martins, and J. Gomes, "Paraben Compounds—Part I: An Overview of Their Characteristics, Detection, and Impacts," *Applied Sciences* 2021, 11 (2021): 2307, https://doi.org/10.3390/app11052307.
4. US Food and Drug Administration, "Perchlorate Questions and Answers," accessed June 5, 2025, https://www.fda.gov/food/environmental-contaminants-food/perchlorate-questions-and-answers.
5. M. Jaishankar, T. Tseten, N. Anbalagan, B. B. Mathew, and K. N. Beeregowda, "Toxicity, Mechanism and Health Effects of Some Heavy Metals," *Interdisciplinary Toxicology* 7, no. 2 (2014): 60–72, https://doi.org/10.2478/intox-2014–0009.
6. European Environment Agency, "Emerging Chemical Risks in Europe—'PFAS,'" updated May 25, 2023, https://www.eea.europa.eu/publications/emerging-chemical-risks-in-europe/emerging-chemical-risks-in-europe.
7. P. Fenichel, N. Chevalier, and F. Brucker-Davis, "Bisphenol A: An Endocrine and Metabolic Disruptor," *Annales d'endocrinologie* 74, no. 3 (2013): 211–20, https://doi.org/10.1016/j.ando.2013.04.002.
8. "EWG's Guide to Sunscreens," Environmental Working Group, accessed June 5, 2025, https://www.ewg.org/sunscreen/report/the-trouble-with-sunscreen-chemicals/.
9. "EWG's Shopper's Guide to Pesticides in Produce," Environmental Working Group, accessed June 5, 2025, https://www.ewg.org/foodnews/full-list.php.
10. A. Gonsioroski, V. E. Mourikes, and J. A. Flaws, "Endocrine Disruptors in Water and Their Effects on the Reproductive System," *International Journal of Molecular Sciences* 21, no. 6 (2020): 1929, https://doi.org/10.3390/ijms21061929.
11. H. Yadav, M. R. H. Khan, M. Quadir, K. A. Rusch, P. P. Mondal, M. Orr, E. G. Xu, and S. M. Iskander, "Cutting Boards: An Overlooked Source of Microplastics in Human Food?" *Environmental Science & Technology* 57, no. 22 (2023): 8225–35, https://doi.org/10.1021/acs.est.3c00924.
12. "Exposures Add Up—Survey Results (2004)," Environmental Working Group, published June 15, 2004, http://www.ewg.org/skindeep/2004/06/15/exposures-add-up-survey-results/.

13. "The Inside Story: A Guide to Indoor Air Quality," Environmental Protection Agency, accessed June 5, 2025, https://www.epa.gov/indoor-air-quality-iaq/inside-story-guide-indoor-air-quality?utm_source=chatgpt.com.

Appendix C: Consider Adaptogens and Other Nutritional Compounds

1. A. Panossian and G. Wikman, "Effects of Adaptogens on the Central Nervous System and the Molecular Mechanisms Associated with Their Stress-Protective Activity," *Pharmaceuticals (Basel)* 3, no. 1 (2010): 188–224, https://doi.org/10.3390/ph3010188.
2. A. Panossian and G. Wikman, "Effects of Adaptogens on the Central Nervous System and the Molecular Mechanisms Associated with Their Stress-Protective Activity," *Pharmaceuticals (Basel)* 3, no. 1 (2010):188–224, https://doi.org/10.3390/ph3010188.
3. D. Winston and S. Maimes, *Adaptogens: Herbs for Strength, Stamina, and Stress Relief—Updated and Expanded*, 2nd ed. (Healing Arts Press, 2019).
4. K. Chandrasekhar, J. Kapoor, and S. Anishetty, "A Prospective, Randomized Double-Blind, Placebo-Controlled Study of Safety and Efficacy of a High-Concentration Full-Spectrum Extract of Ashwagandha Root in Reducing Stress and Anxiety in Adults," *Indian Journal of Psychological Medicine* 34, no. 3 (2012):255–62.
5. M. A. Pratte, K. B. Nanavati, V, Young, C. P. Morley, "An Alternative Treatment for Anxiety: A Systematic Review of Human Trial Results Reported for the Ayurvedic Herb Ashwagandha (*Withania somnifera*)," *Journal of Alternative and Complementary Medicine* 20, no. 12 (2014): 901–8.
6. A. K. Sharma, I. Basu, and S. Singh S. "Efficacy and Safety of Ashwagandha Root Extract in Subclinical Hypothyroid Patients: A Double-Blind, Randomized Placebo-Controlled Trial," *Journal of Alternative and Complementary Medicine* 24, no. 3 (2018): 243–48, https://doi.org/10.1089/acm.2017.0183.
7. S. K. Hung, R. Perry, and E. Ernst, "The Effectiveness and Efficacy of Rhodiola Rosea L.: A Systematic Review of Randomized Clinical Trials," *Phytomedicine* 18, no. 4 (2011): 235–44, https://doi.org/10.1016/j.phymed.2010.08.014.
8. N. M. Arring, D. Millstine, L. A. Marks, and L. M. Nail, "Ginseng as a Treatment for Fatigue: A Systematic Review," *Journal of Alternative and Complementary Medicine* 24 , no. 7 (2018): 624–33, https://doi.org/10.1089/acm.2017.0361.

9. M. Jakaria, M. E. Haque, J. Kim, D. Y. Cho, I.S. Kim, and D. K. Choi, "Active Ginseng Components in Cognitive Impairment: Therapeutic Potential and Prospects for Delivery and Clinical Study," *Oncotarget* 9, no. 71 (2018): 33601–20, https://doi.org/10.18632/oncotarget.26035.
10. S. Lee and D. K. Rhee, "Effects of Ginseng on Stress-Related Depression, Anxiety, and the Hypothalamic-Pituitary-Adrenal Axis," *Journal of Ginseng Research* 41, no. 4 (2017): 589–94, https://doi.org/10.1016/j.jgr.2017.01.010.
11. N. Jamshidi and M. M. Cohen, "The Clinical Efficacy and Safety of Tulsi in Humans: a Systematic Review of the Literature," *Evidence-Based Complementary and Alternative Medicine* 2017: 9217567, https://doi.org/10.1155/2017/9217567.
12. Palmiero Monteleone, Lucia Beinat, Carla Tanzillo, Mario Maj, Dargut Kemali, "Effects of Phosphatidylserine on the Neuroendocrine Response to Physical Stress in Humans," *Neuroendocrinology* 52, no. 3 (1990): 243–48, https://doi.org/10.1159/000125593l; P. Monteleone, M. Maj, L. Beinat, M. Natale, and D. Kemali, "Blunting by Chronic Phosphatidylserine Administration of the Stress-Induced Activation of the Hypothalamo-Pituitary-Adrenal Axis in Healthy Men," *European Journal of Clinical Pharmacology* 42, no. 4 (1992): 385–88.
13. Palmiero Monteleone, Lucia Beinat, Carla Tanzillo, Mario Maj, and Dargut Kemali, "Effects of Phosphatidylserine on the Neuroendocrine Response to Physical Stress in Humans," *Neuroendocrinology* 52, no. 3 (1990): 243–48, https://doi.org/10.1159/000125593; P. Monteleone, M. Maj, L. Beinat, M. Natale, and D. Kemali, "Blunting by Chronic Phosphatidylserine Administration of the Stress-Induced Activation of the Hypothalamo-Pituitary-Adrenal Axis in Healthy Men," *European Journal of Clinical Pharmacology* 42, no. 4 (1992): 385–98.
14. P. Heilmann, J. Heide, S. Hundertmark, and M. Schoneshofer, "Administration of Glycyrrhetinic Acid: Significant Correlation Between Serum Levels and the Cortisol/Cortisone-Ratio in Serum and Urine," *Experimental and Clinical Endocrinology and Diabetes* 107, no. 6 (1999): 370–78.

Index

About the Author

Marina Wright is a functional diagnostic nutrition practitioner and certified integrative nutrition health coach, with a mind-body approach to wellness.

Originally trained in law and economics, Marina spent several years in investment banking before making a career shift. Her passion for holistic health grew as she witnessed firsthand how integrating foundational health practices—such as nutrition, sleep, and exercise—with holistic mind-body techniques is key to achieving optimal physical health and mental well-being.

She holds a bachelor's degree from the Universidad de Navarra in Pamplona, Spain, and has furthered her expertise with certifications from the Institute for Integrative Nutrition and Functional Diagnostic Nutrition. Her additional specialized training includes Mindfulness-Based Stress Reduction (MBSR), somatic stress release, and the gut-brain connection.

Through her online platforms, Marina has taught and empowered thousands of people worldwide to transform their health and well-being through a mind-body approach. Connect with her and join her community on Instagram at @marinawrightwellness for inspiration, tips, and more. To explore her programs, visit www.marinawright.com.

Born and raised in Spain, Marina has also lived and worked in the UK and US for many years. She now resides in Australia with her husband and two children, embracing an active, nature-filled lifestyle and a love of healthy cooking.